Make a Wish

b…
eve… you want.

- Annette White

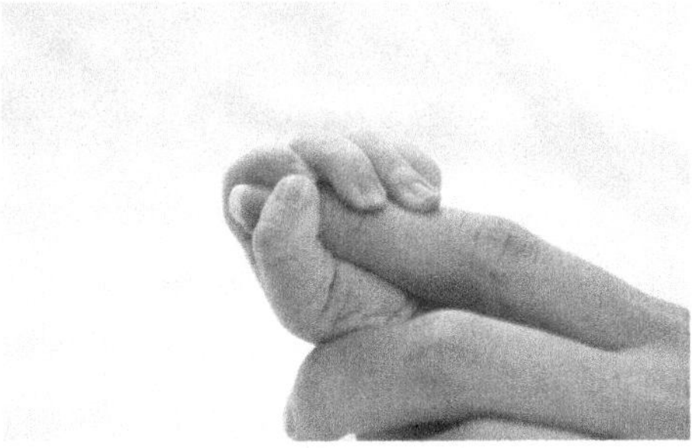

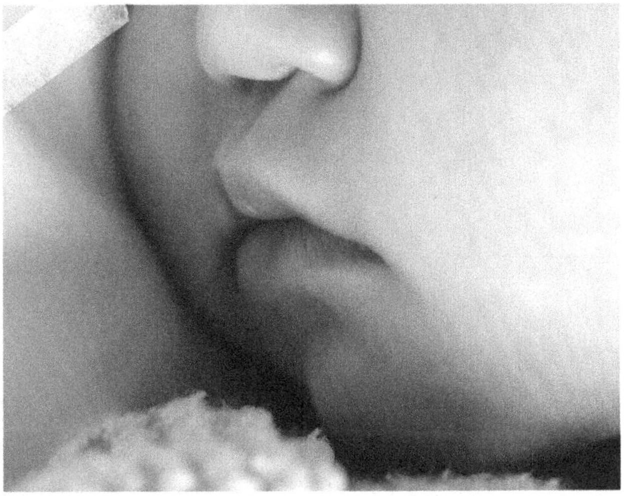

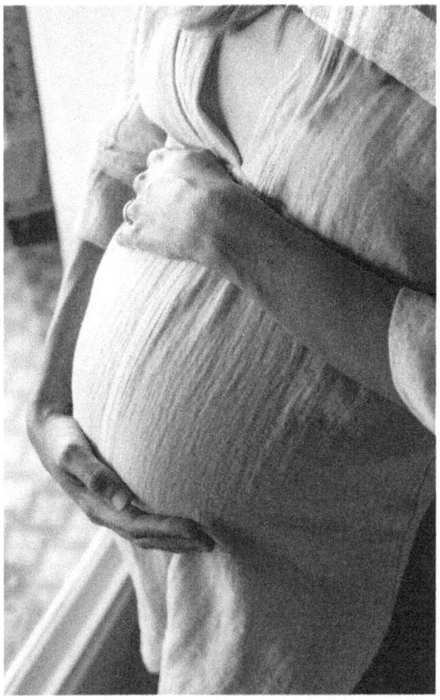

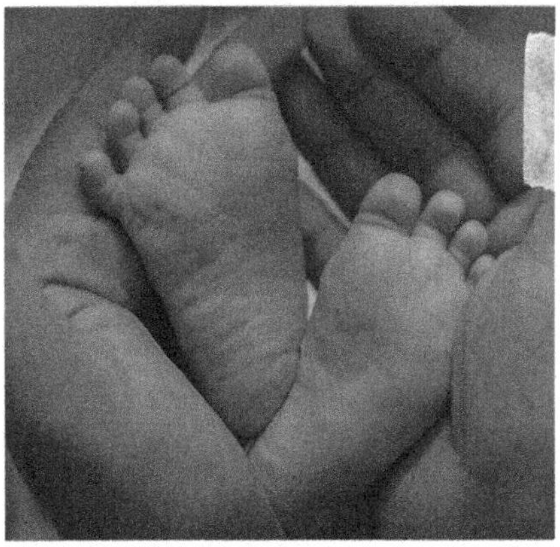

Cut out pictures that represent your dreams, glue them on a board, and visualize your goals daily!

Little Family Publishing

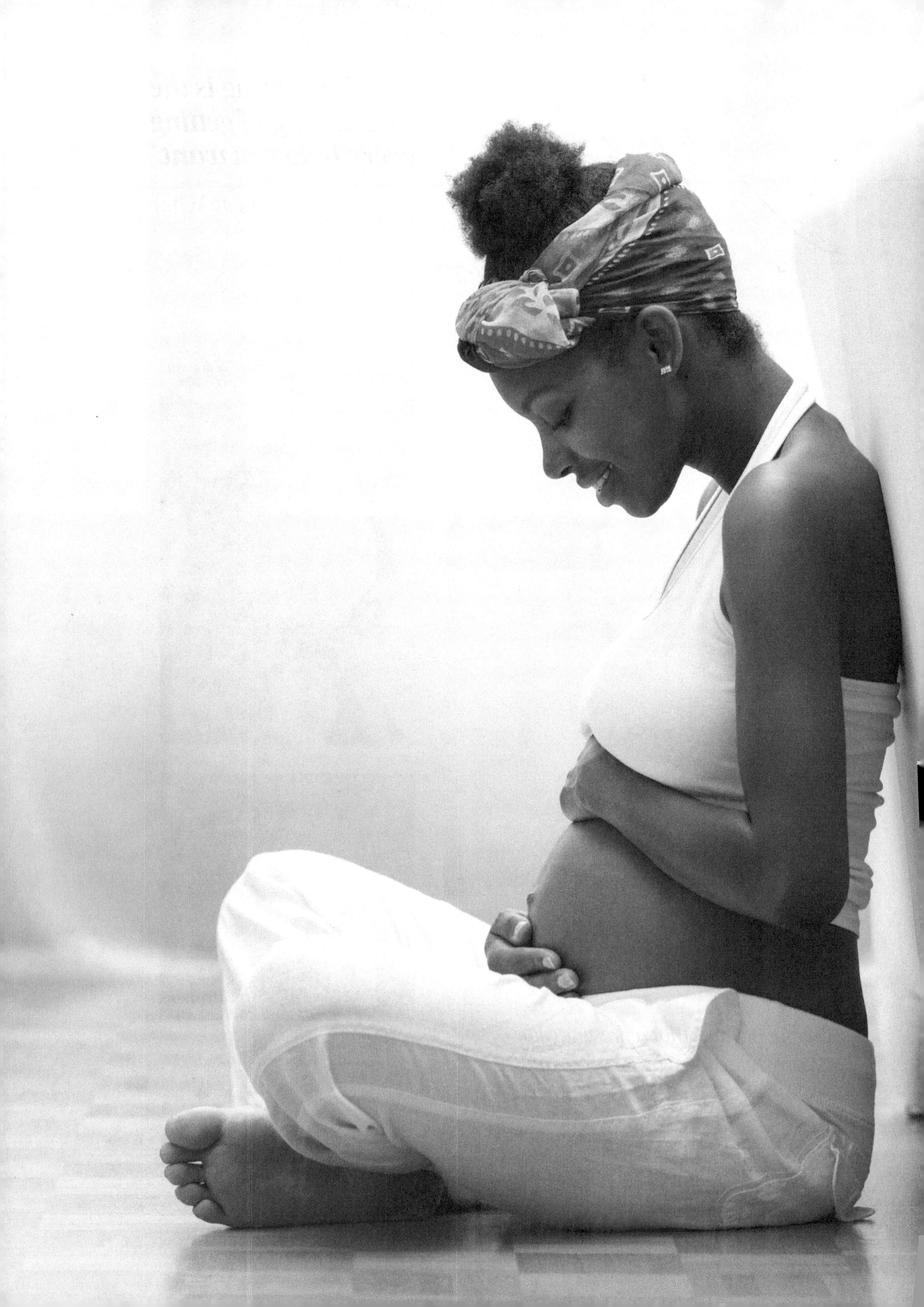

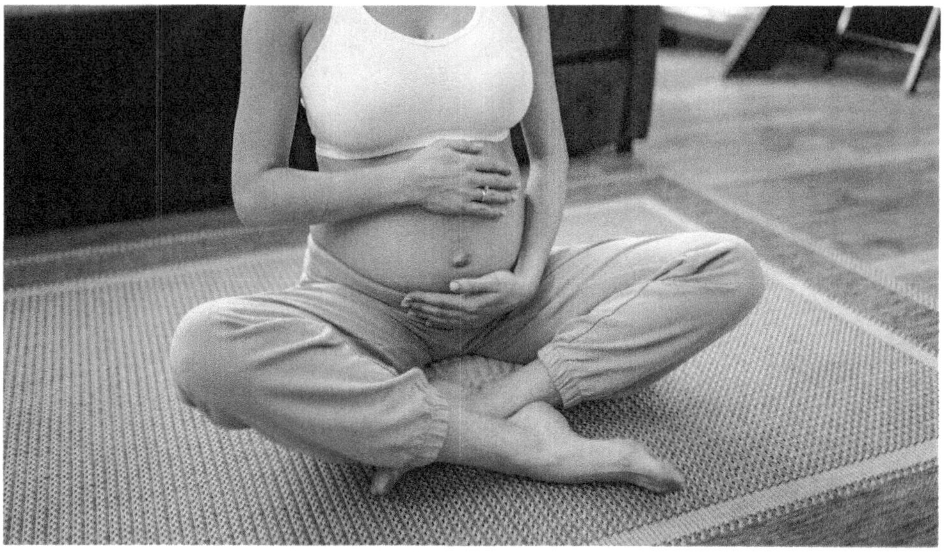
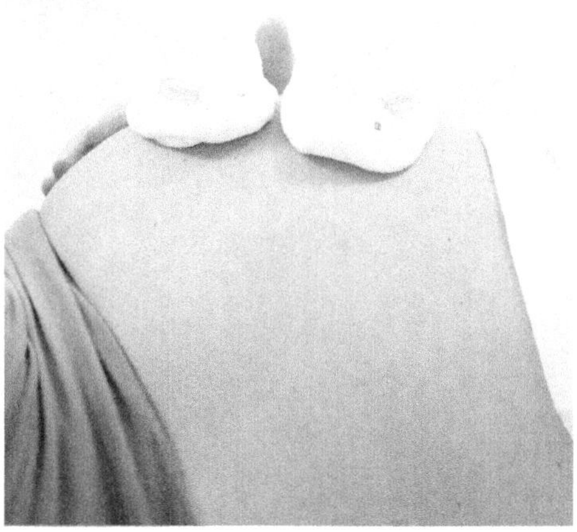
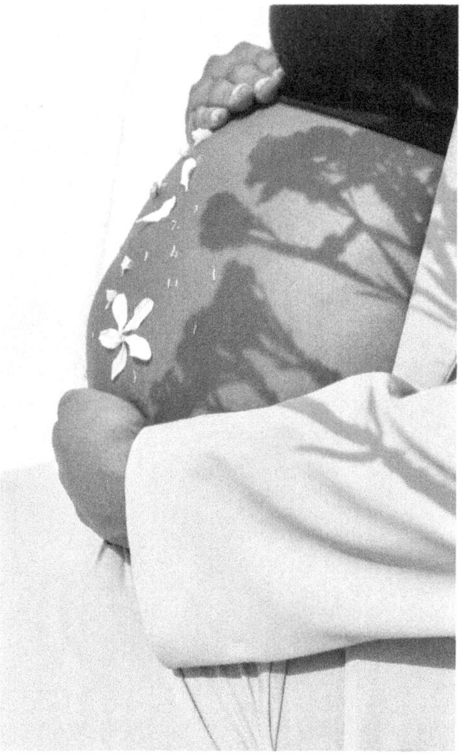
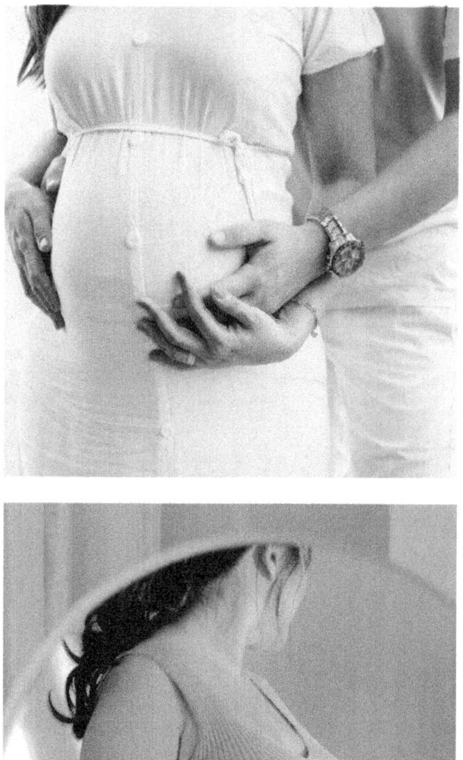
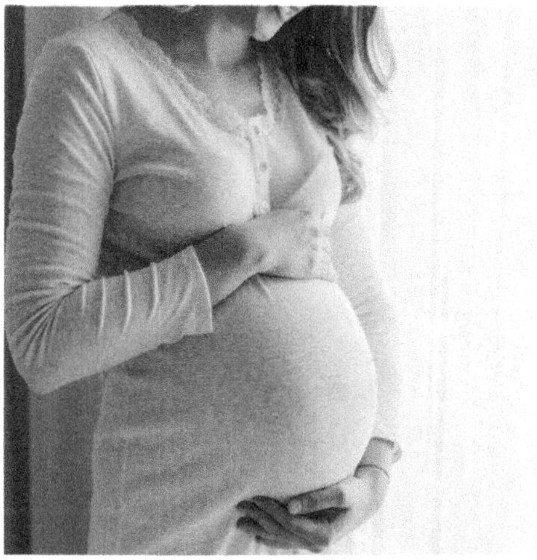
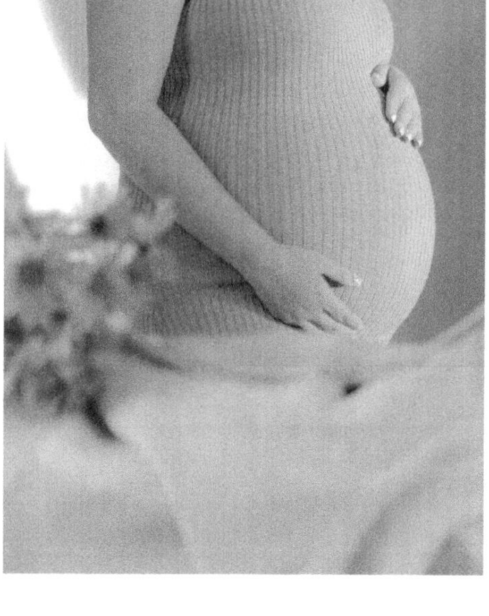
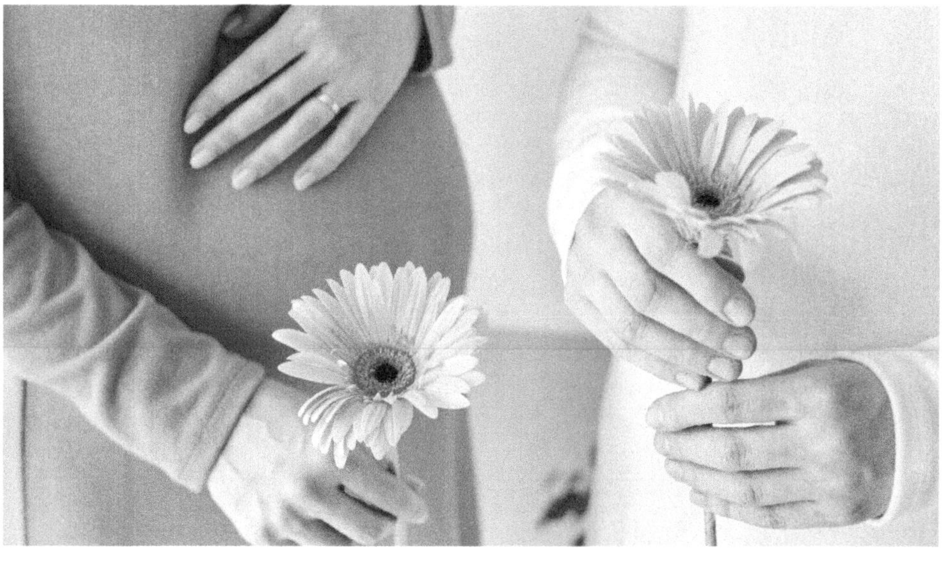

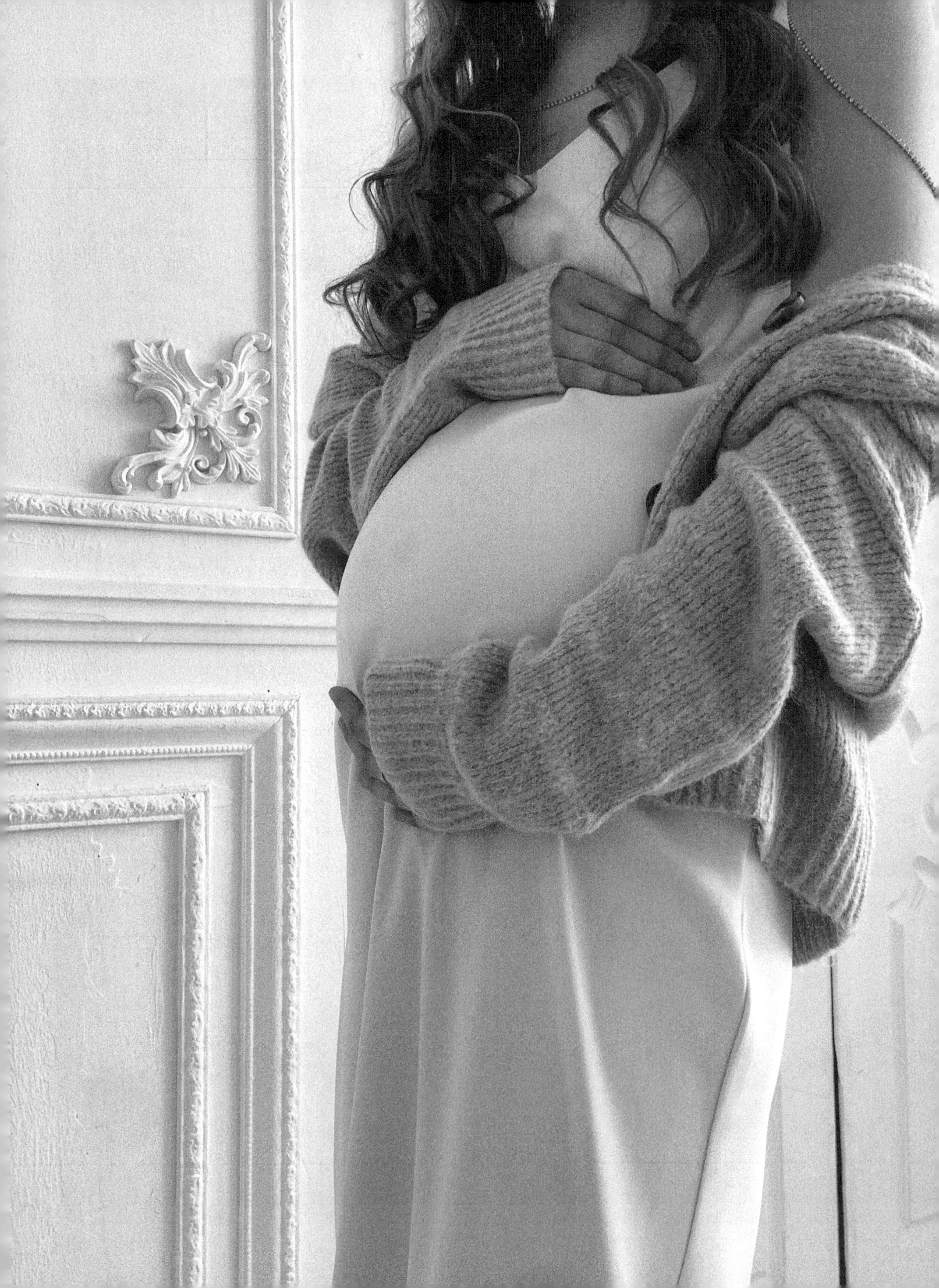

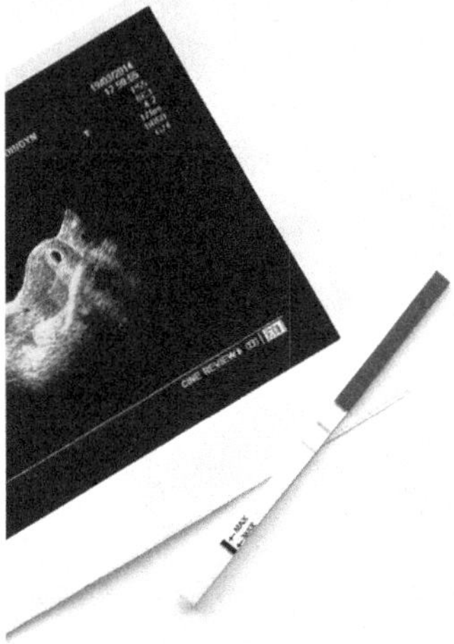

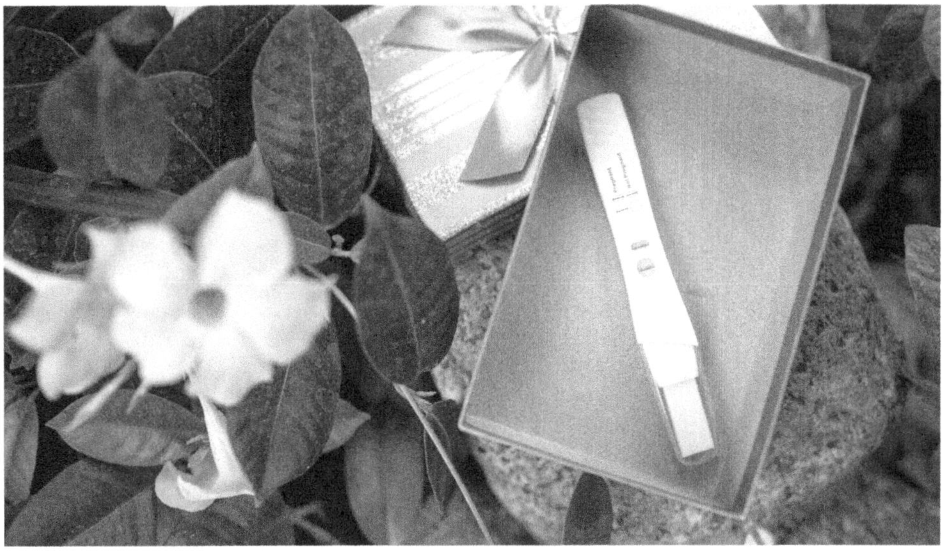

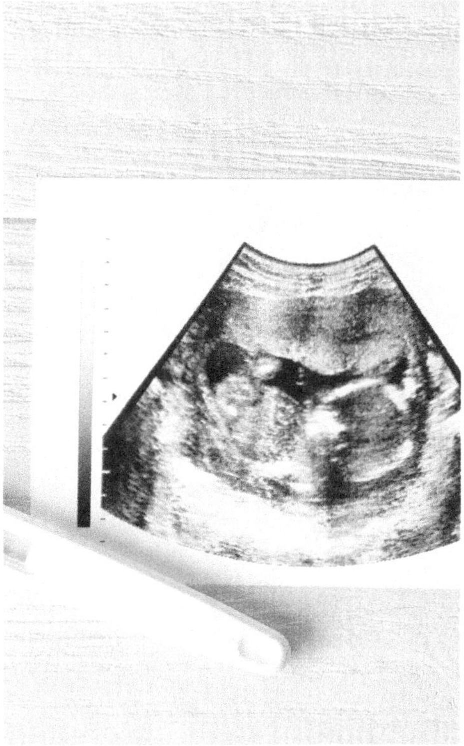

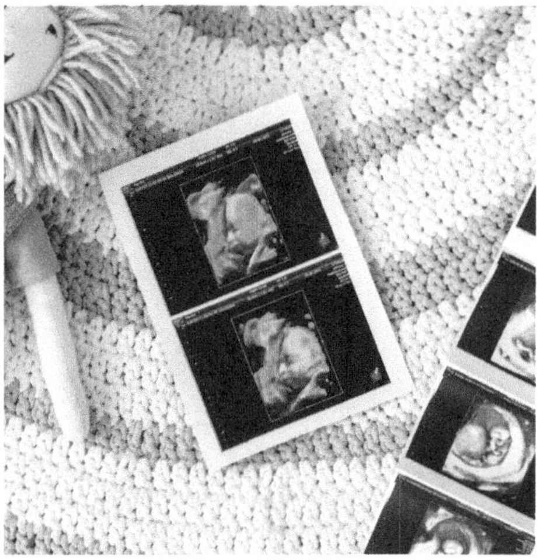

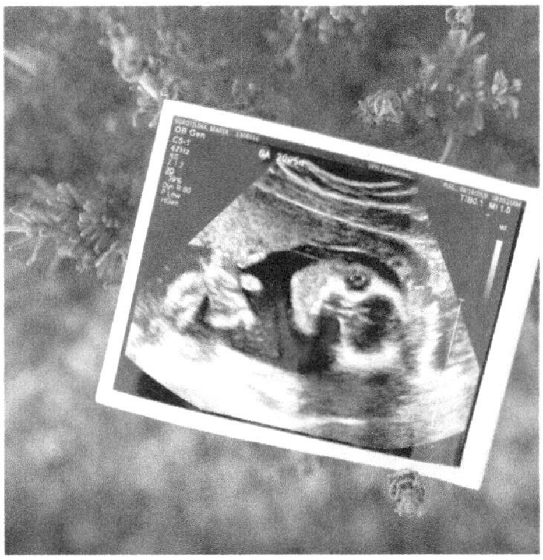

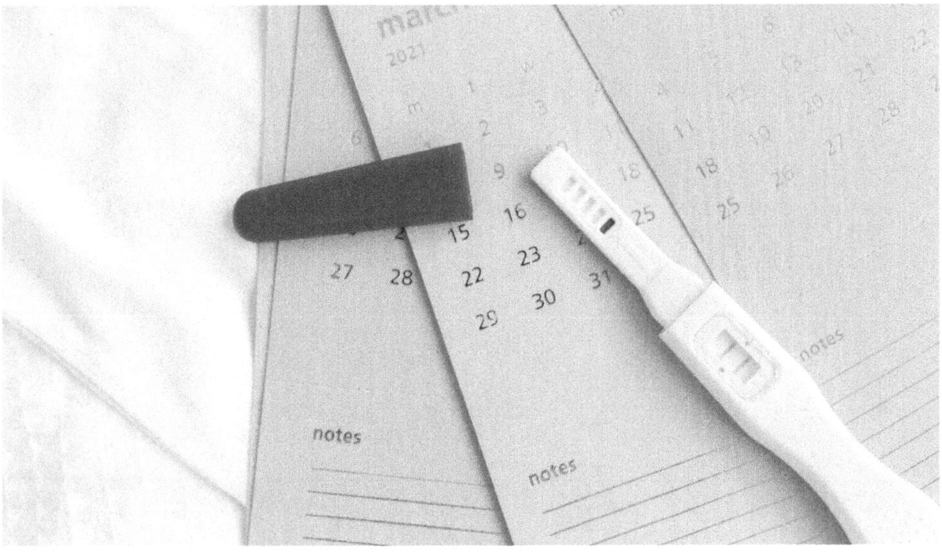
2021
notes
notes
notes

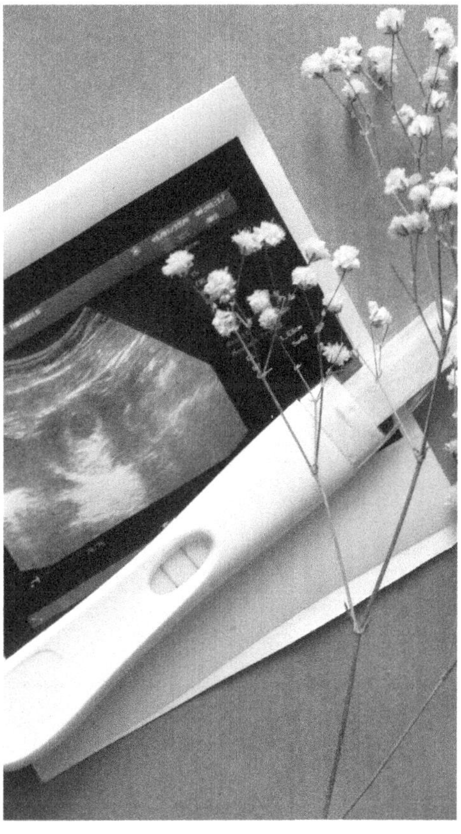

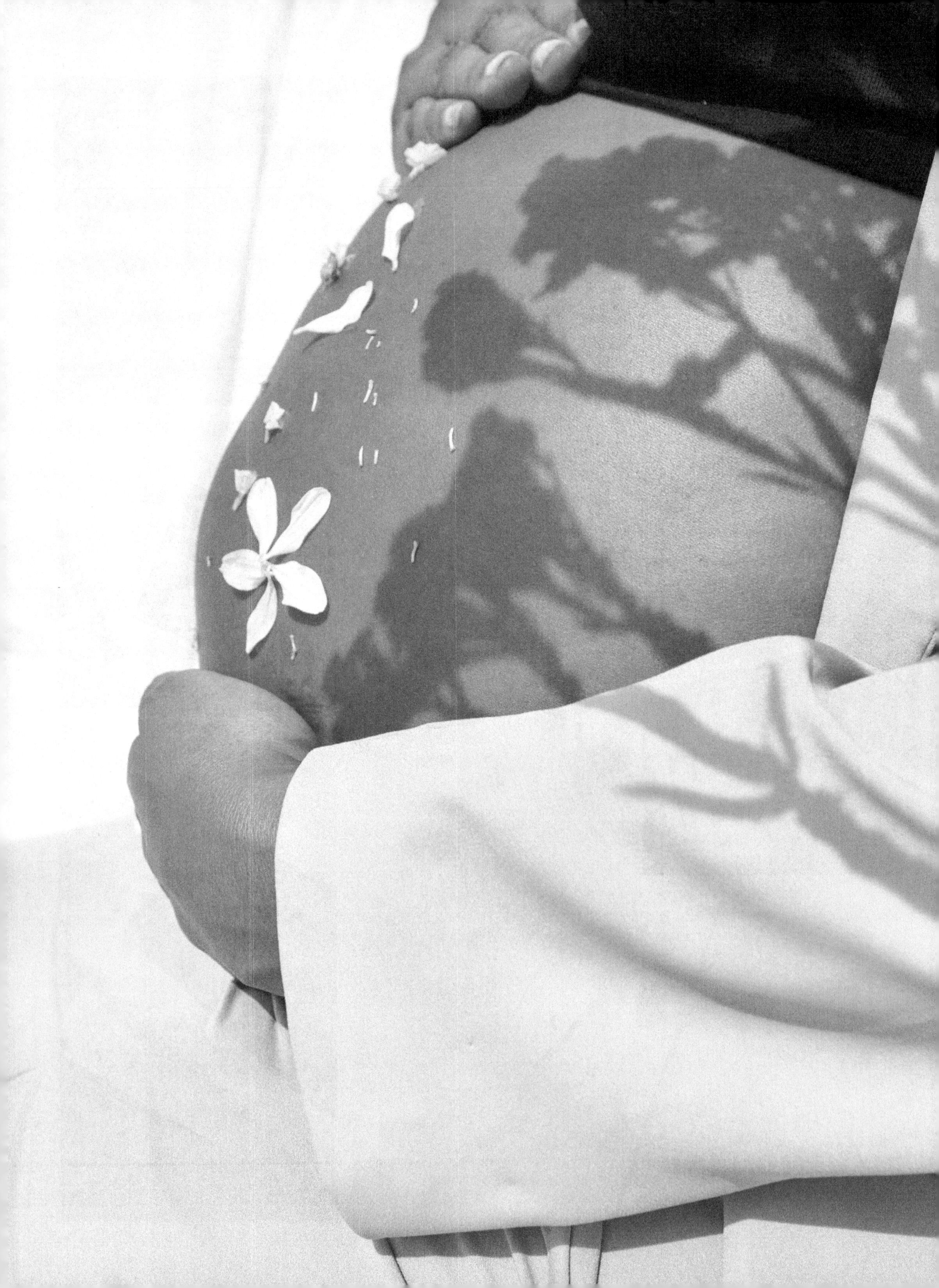

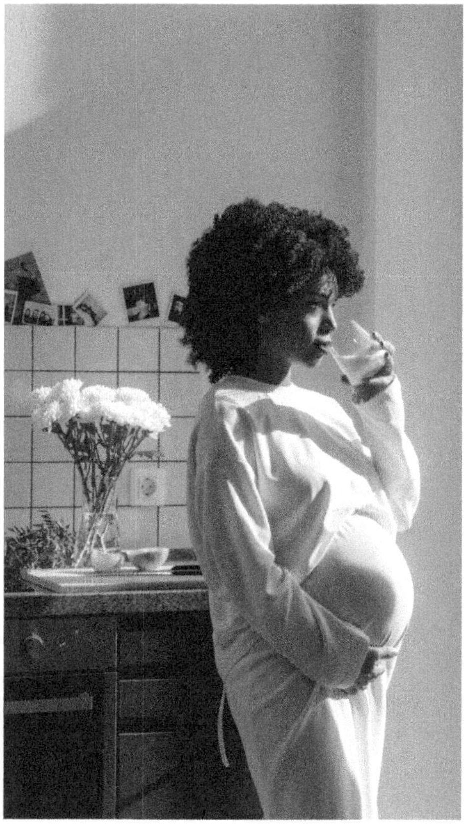
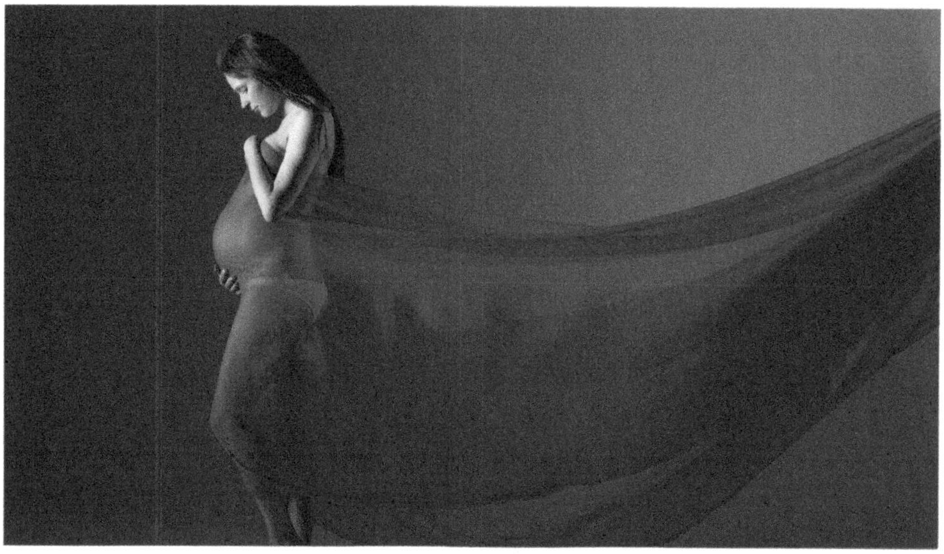
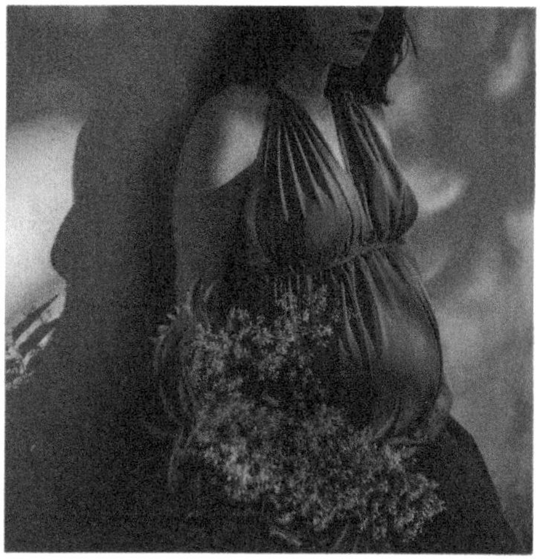
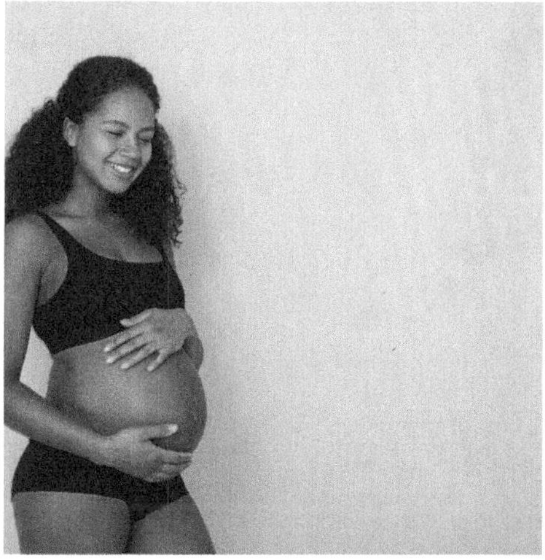
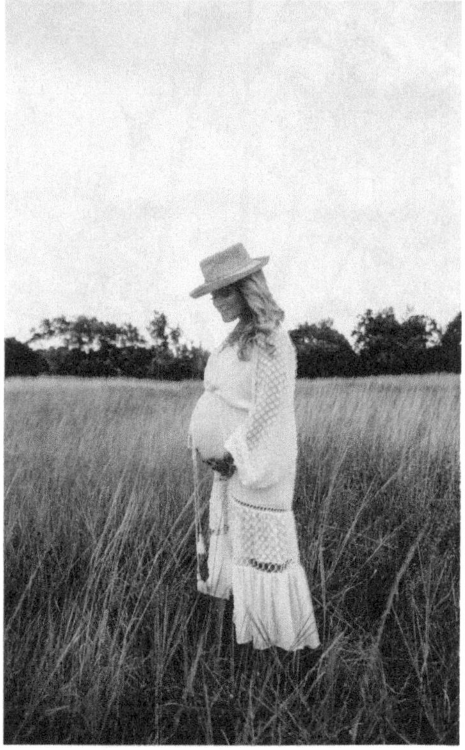
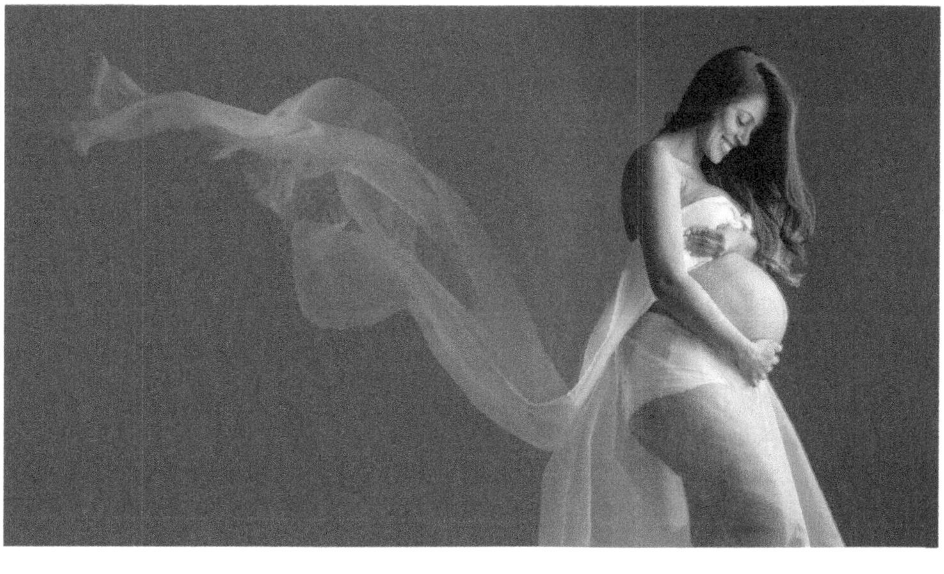
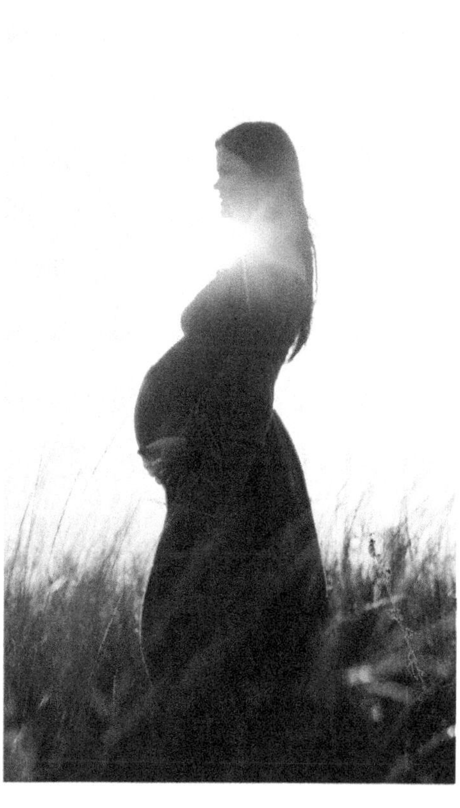

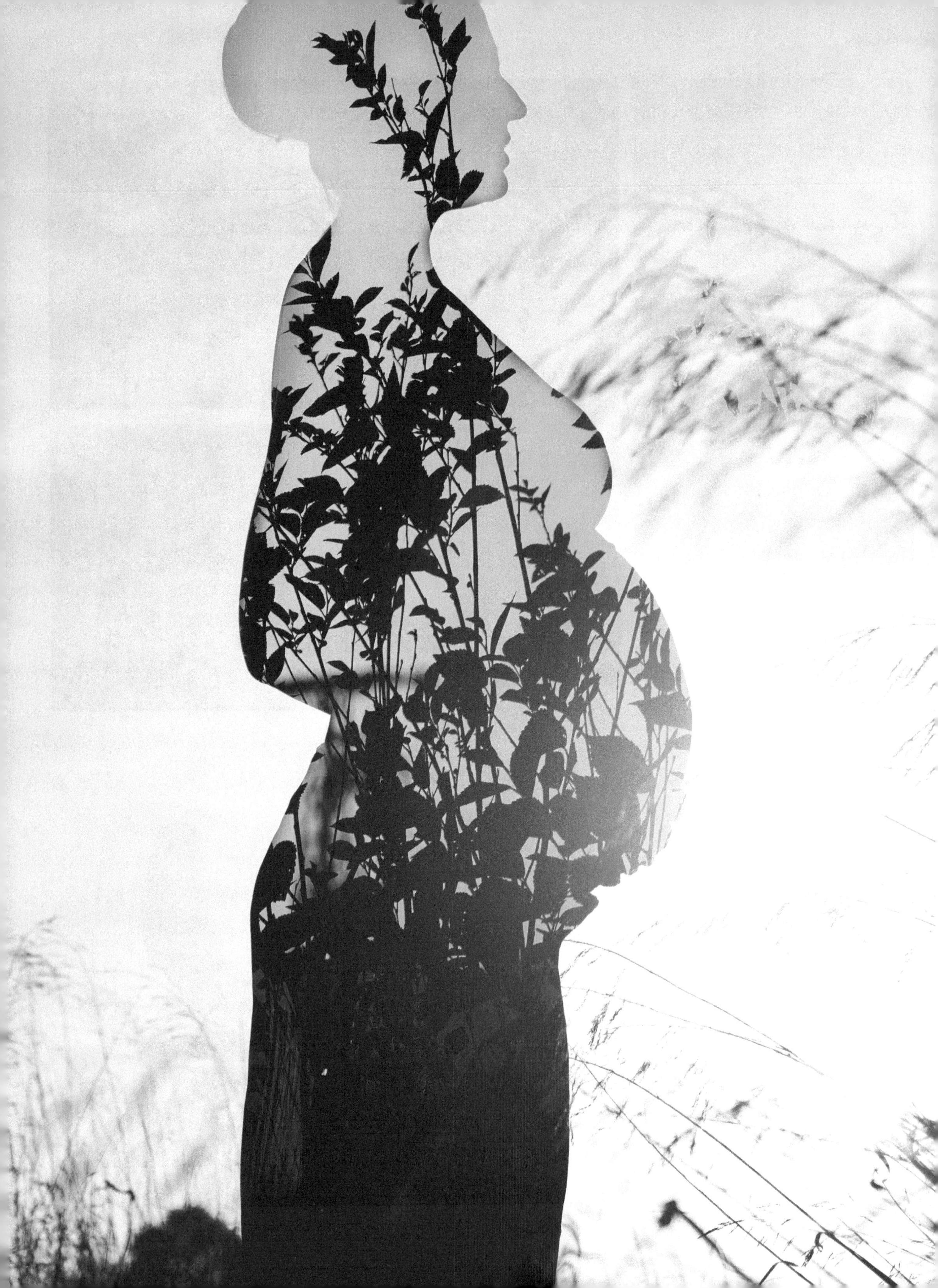

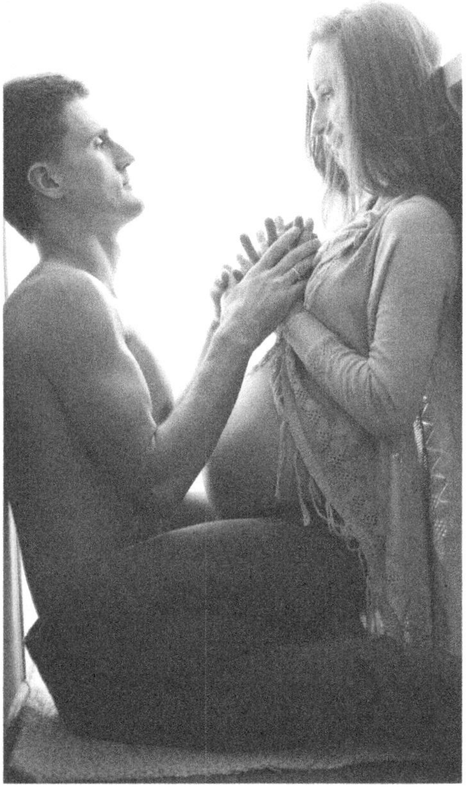
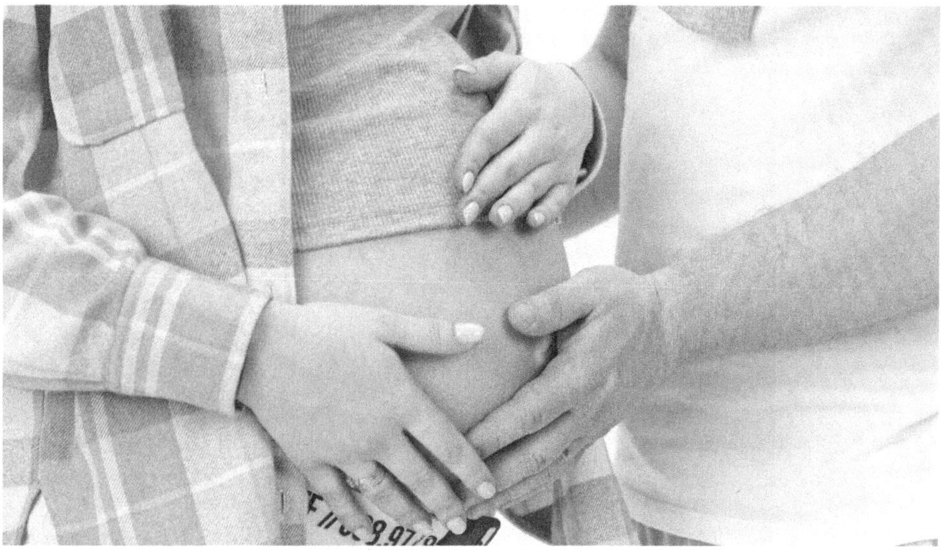
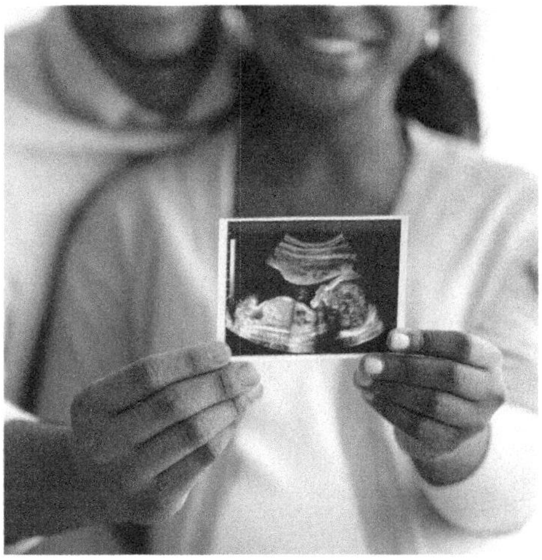
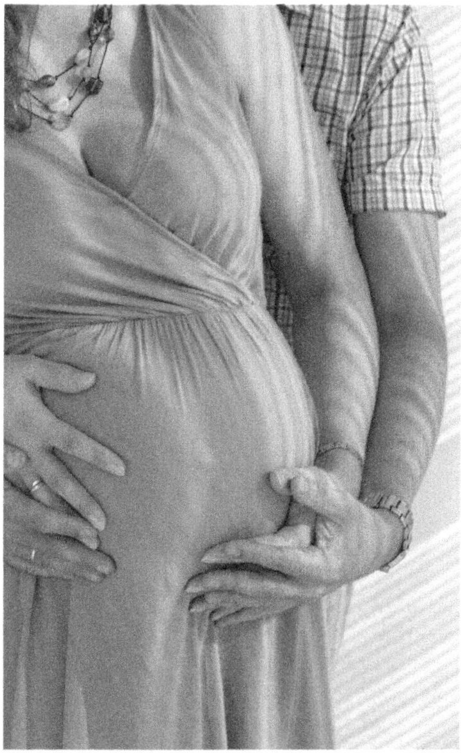
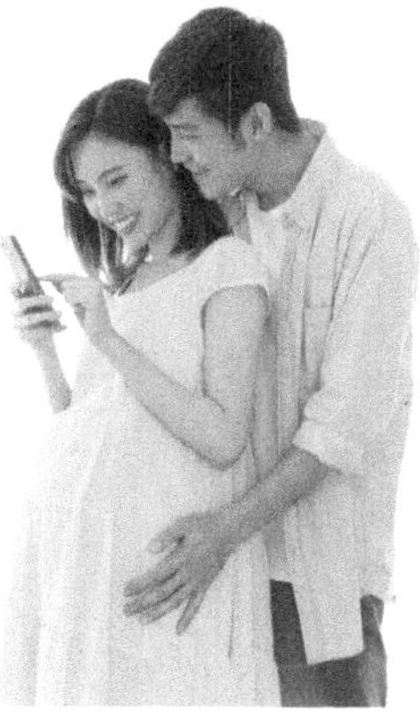
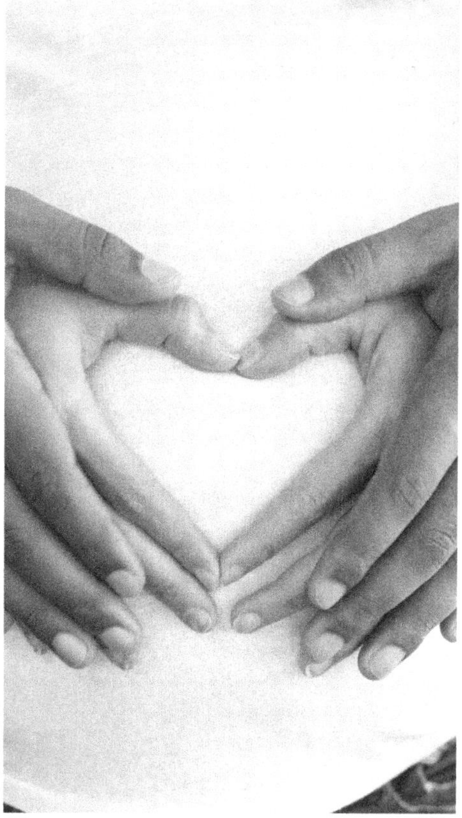
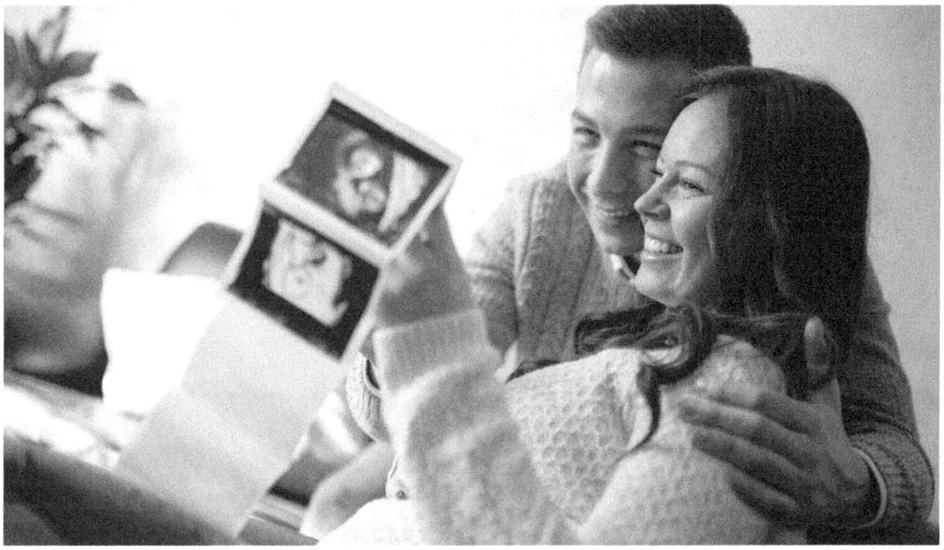

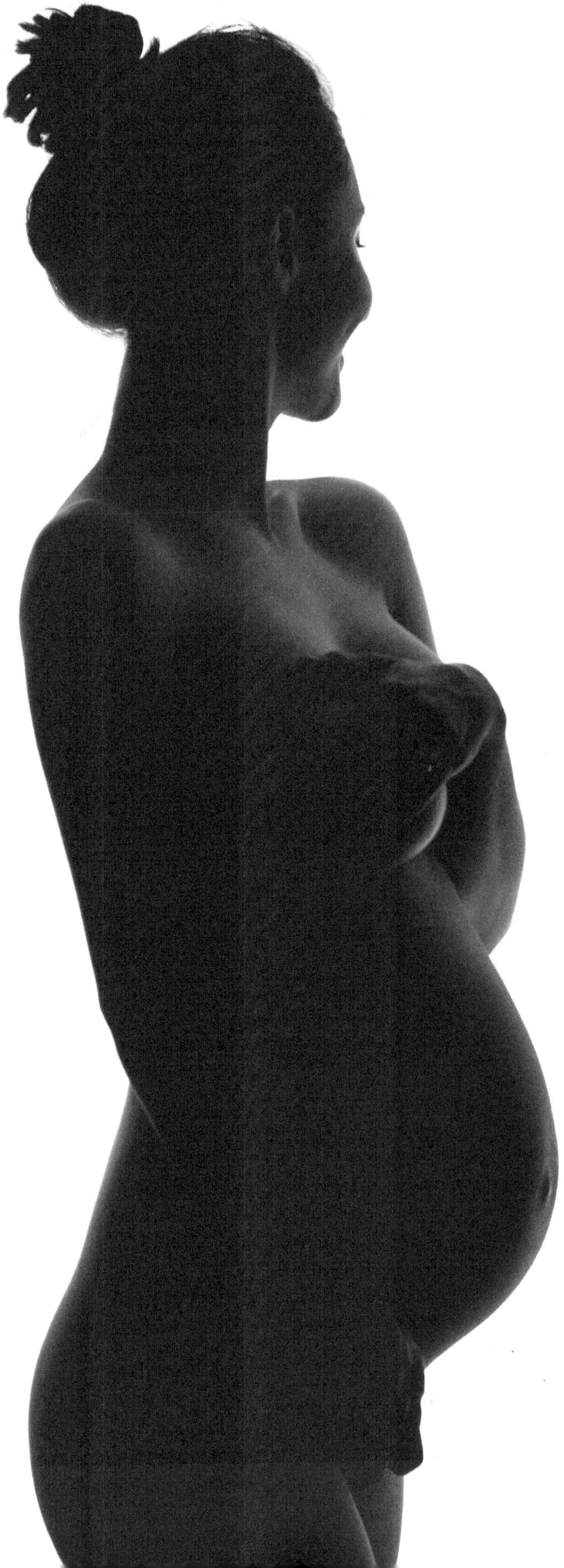

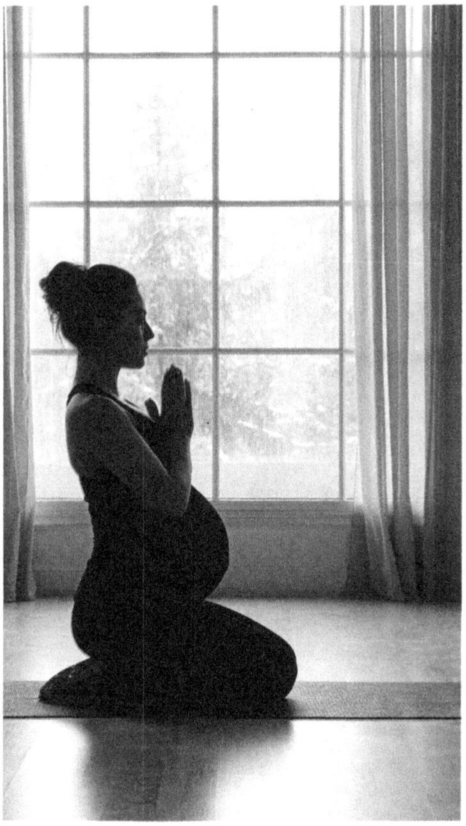

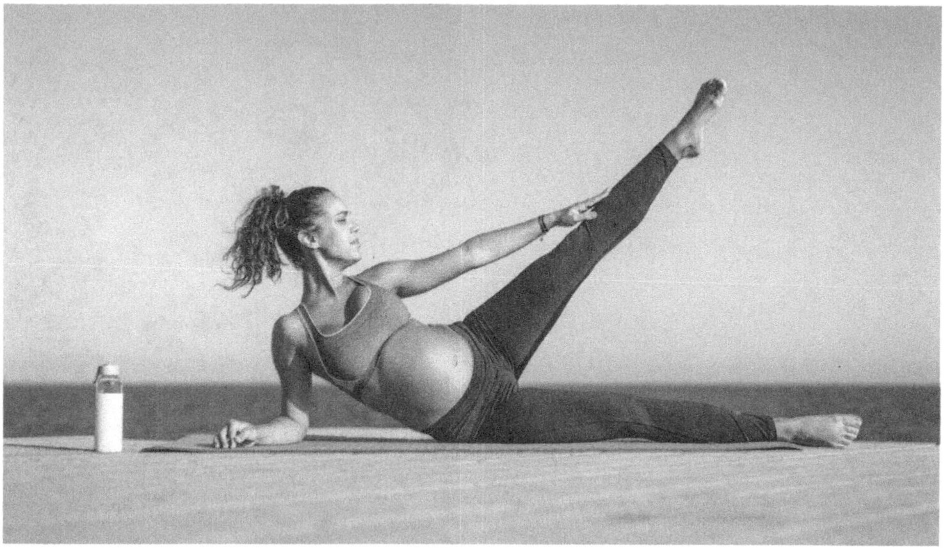

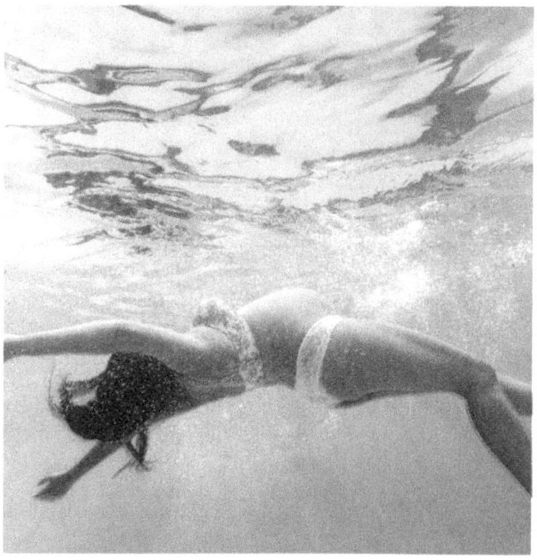

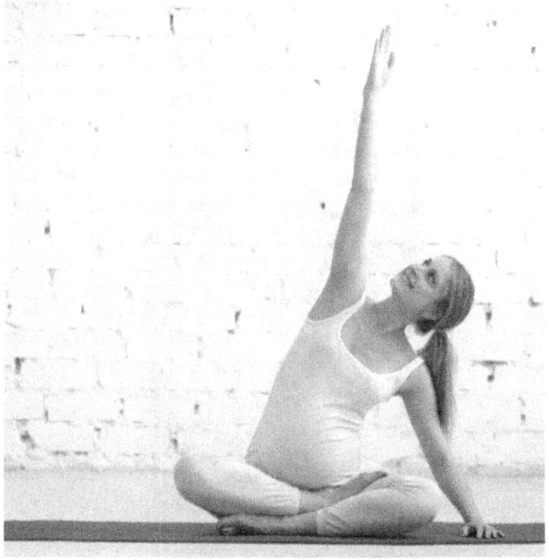

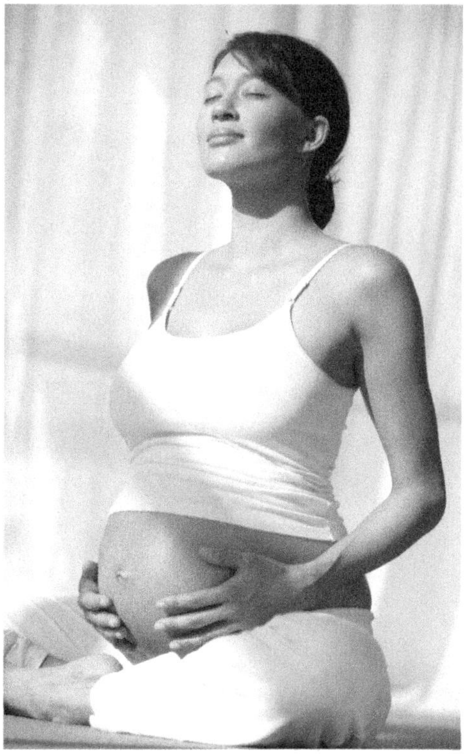

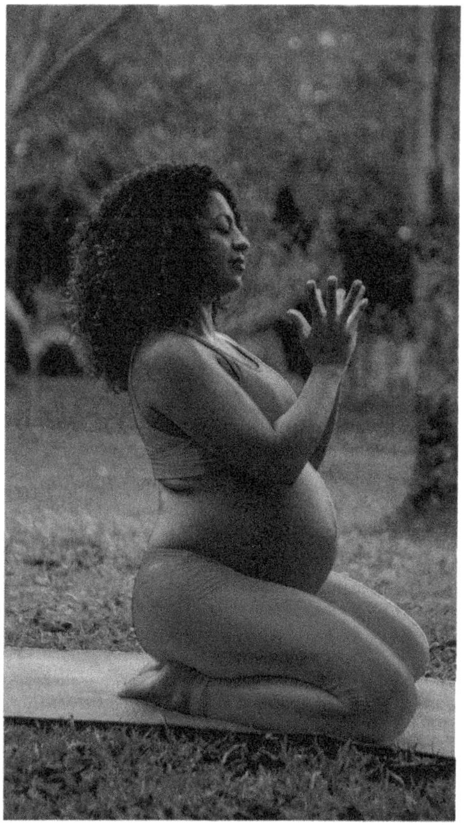

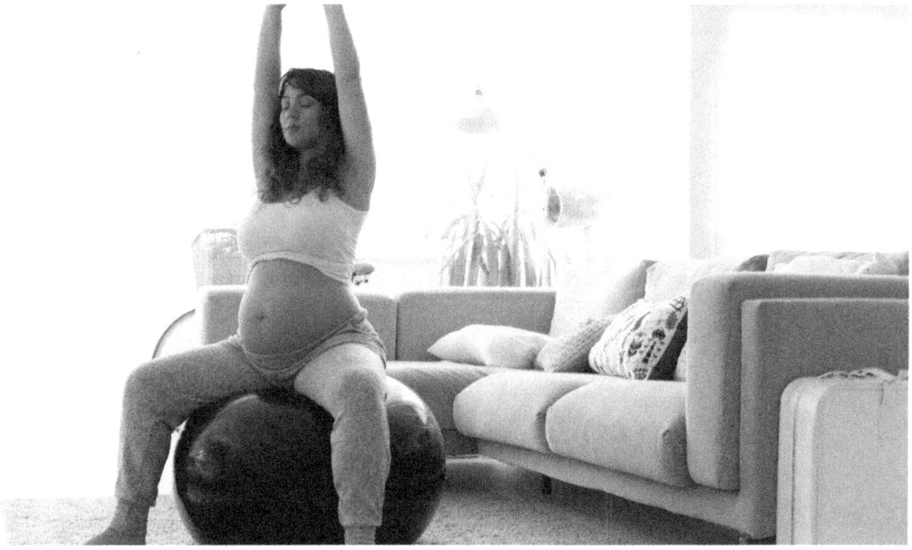

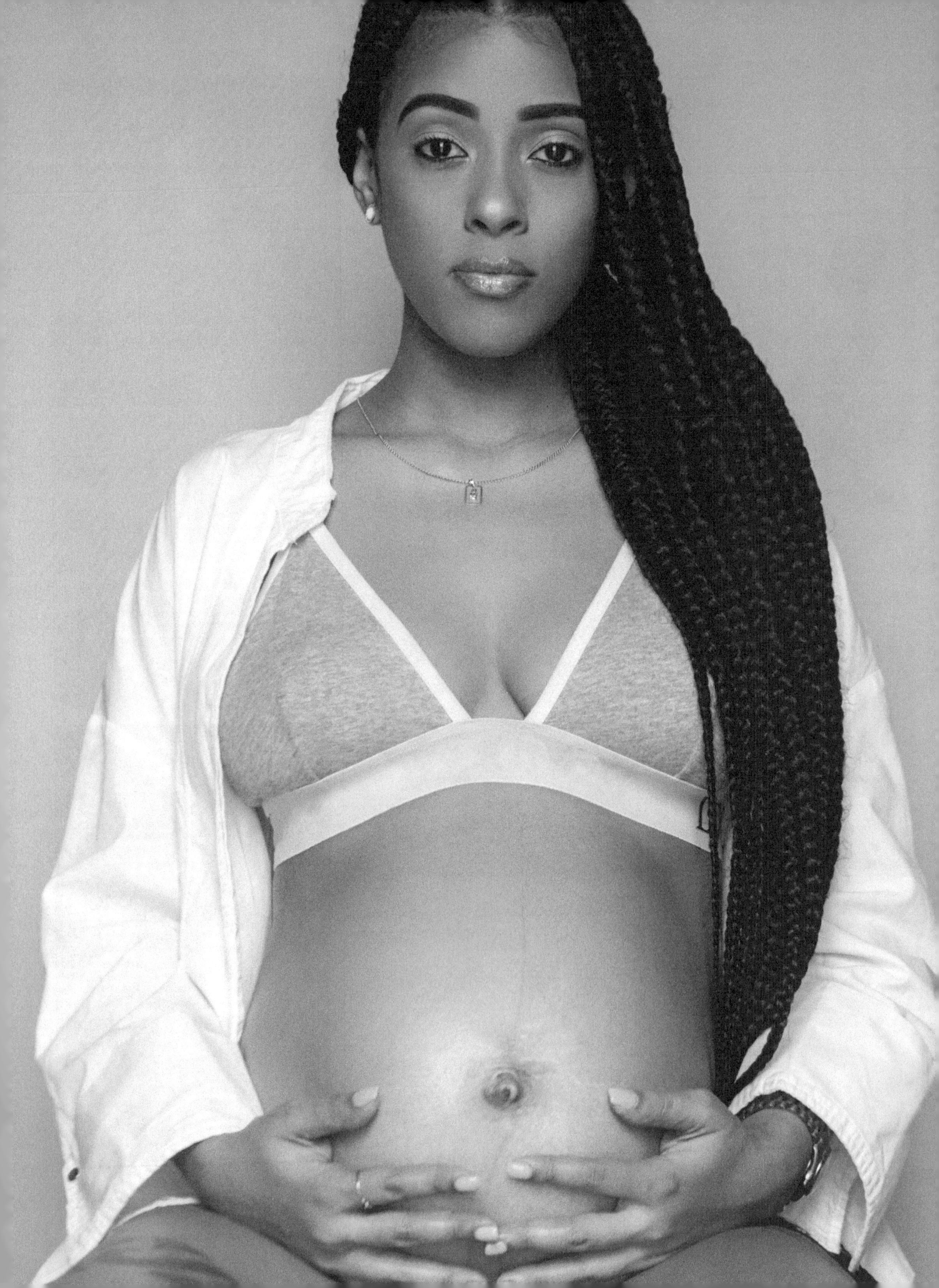

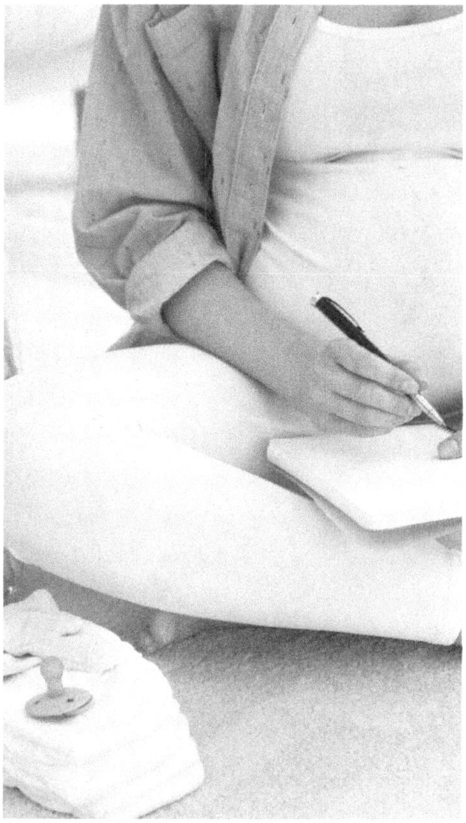
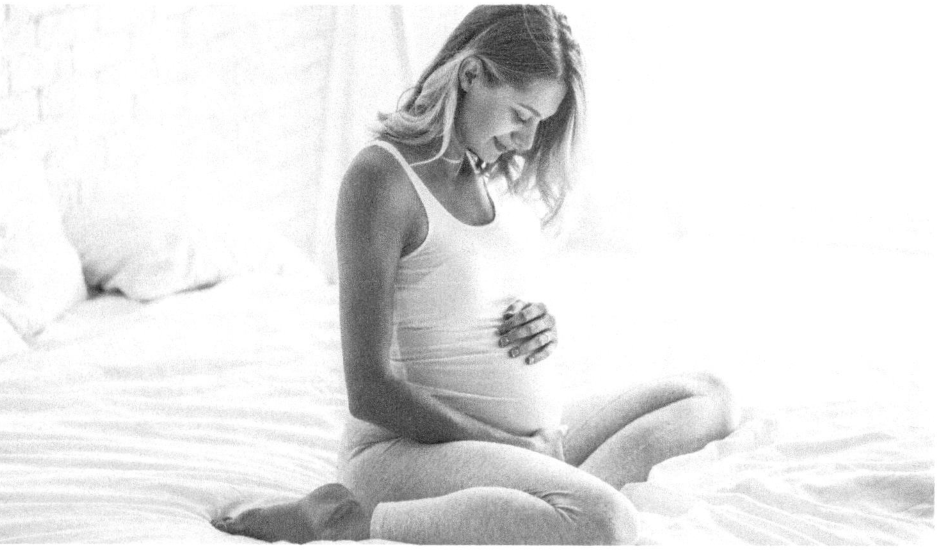
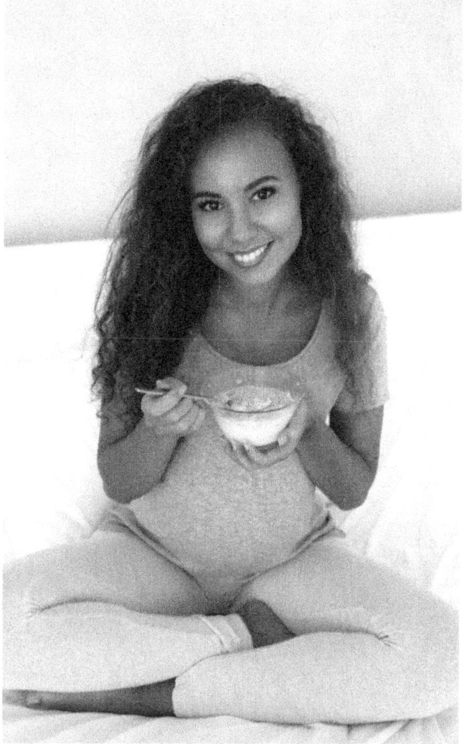
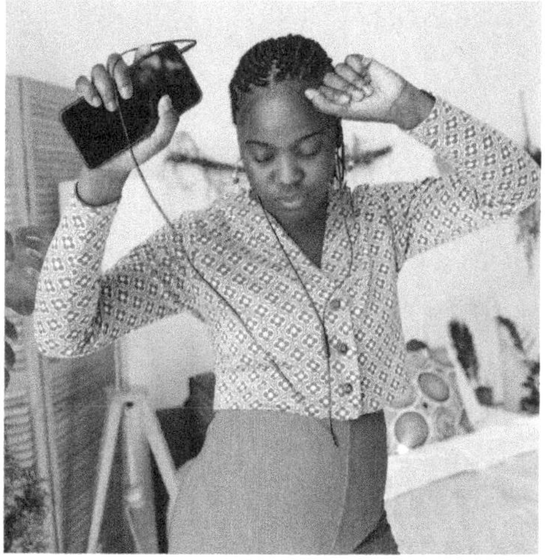
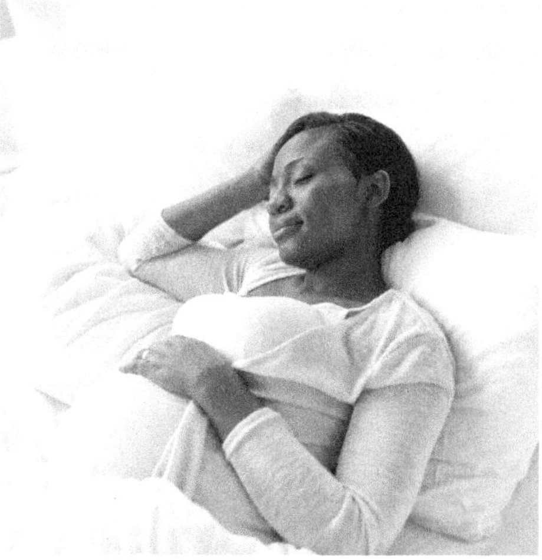
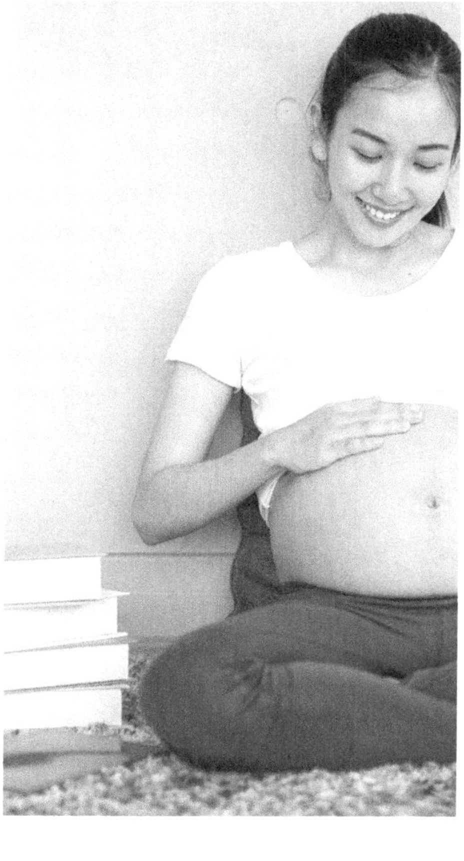
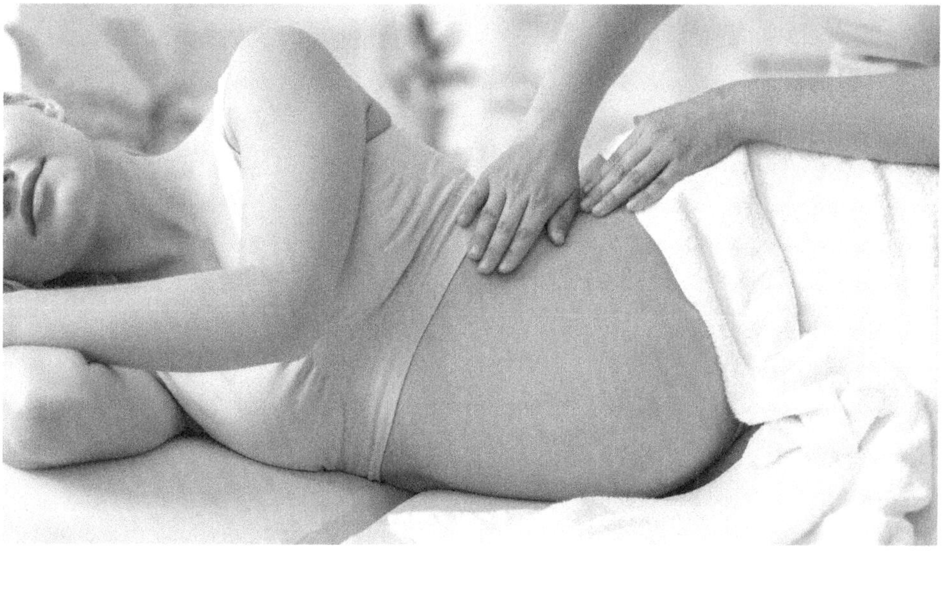

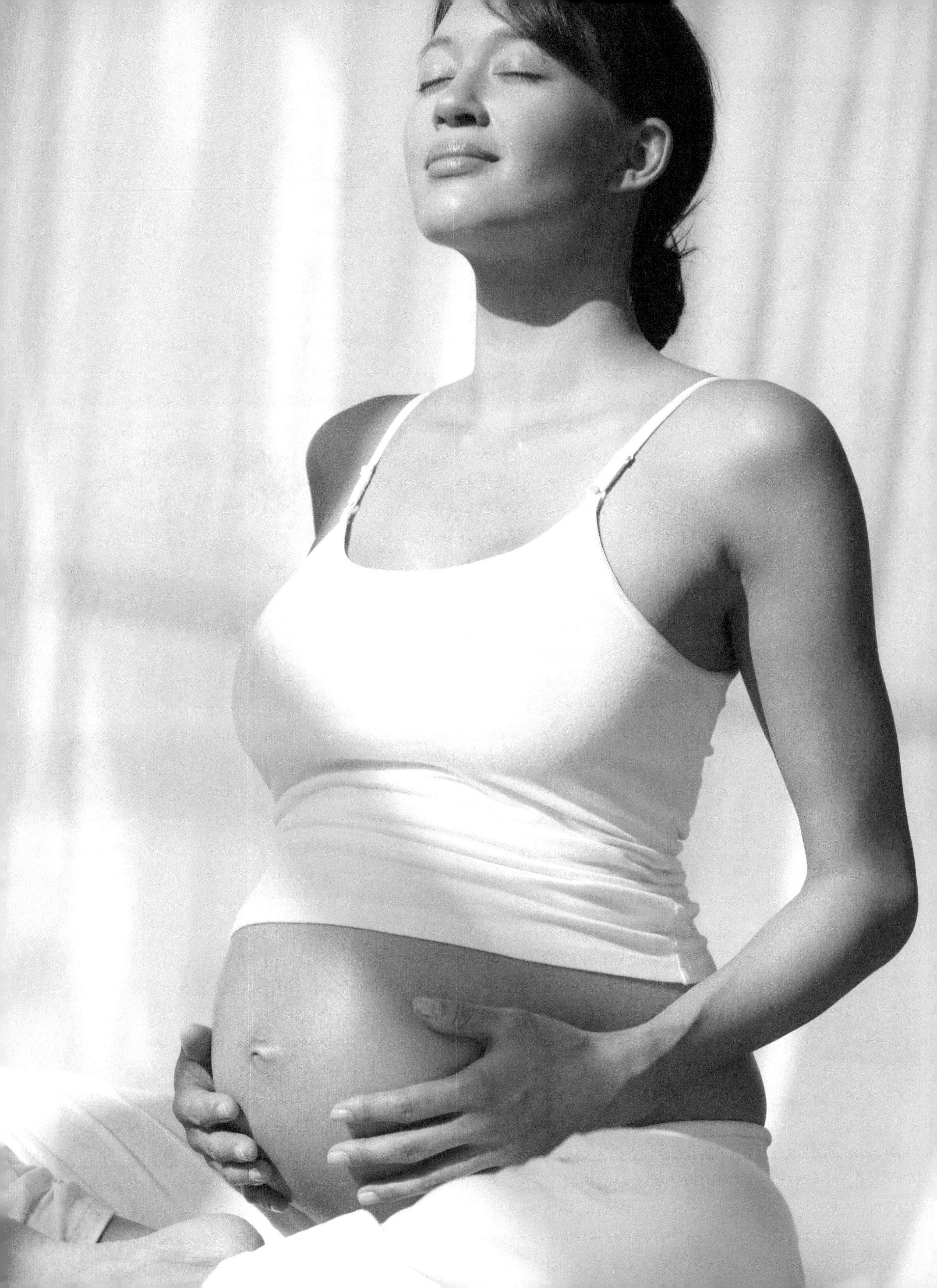

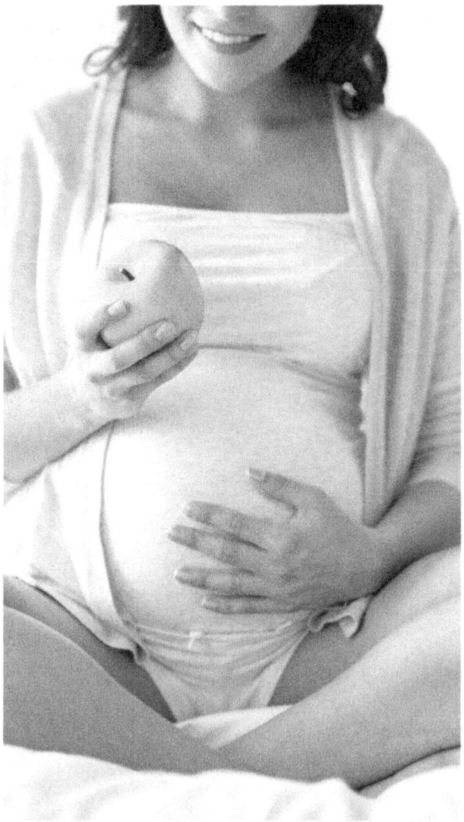
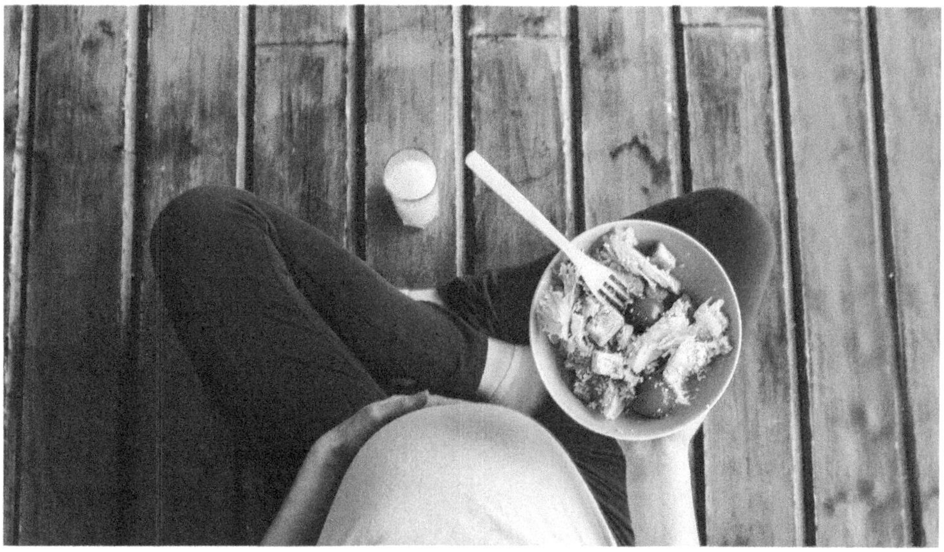
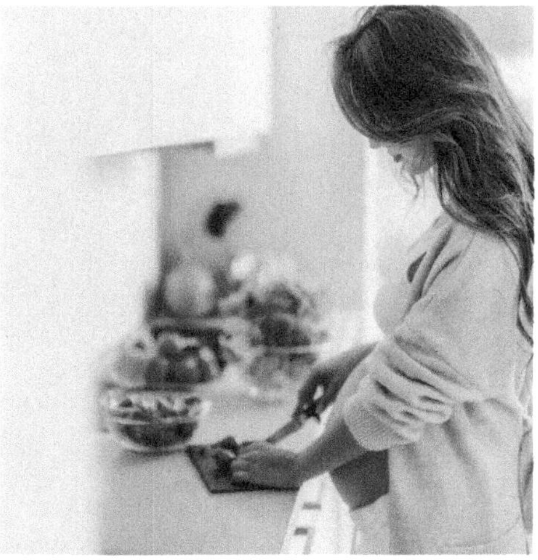
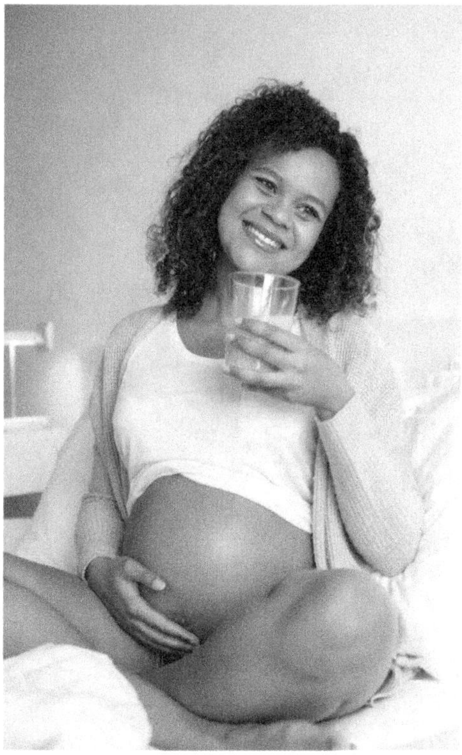
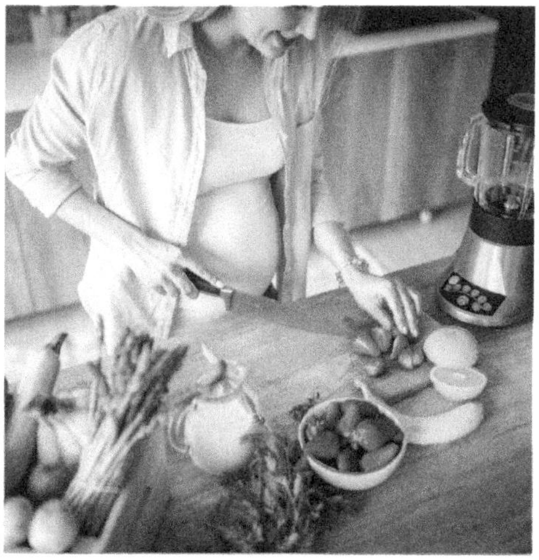
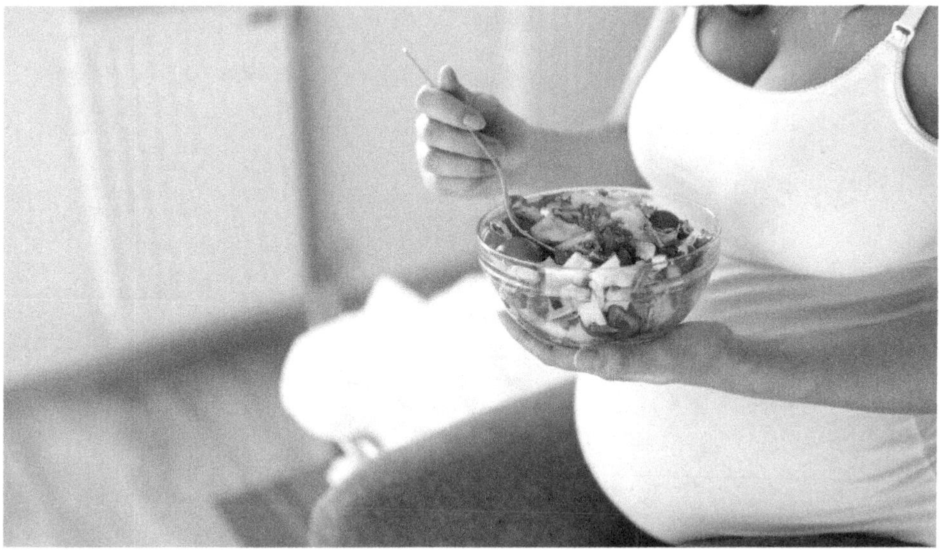
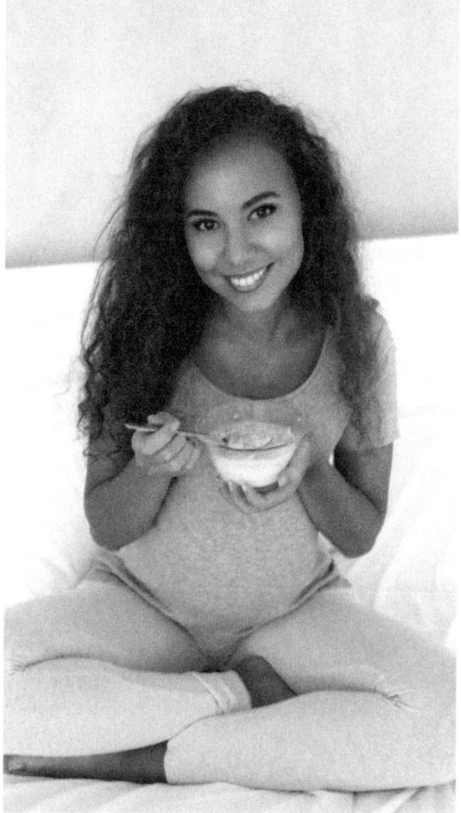

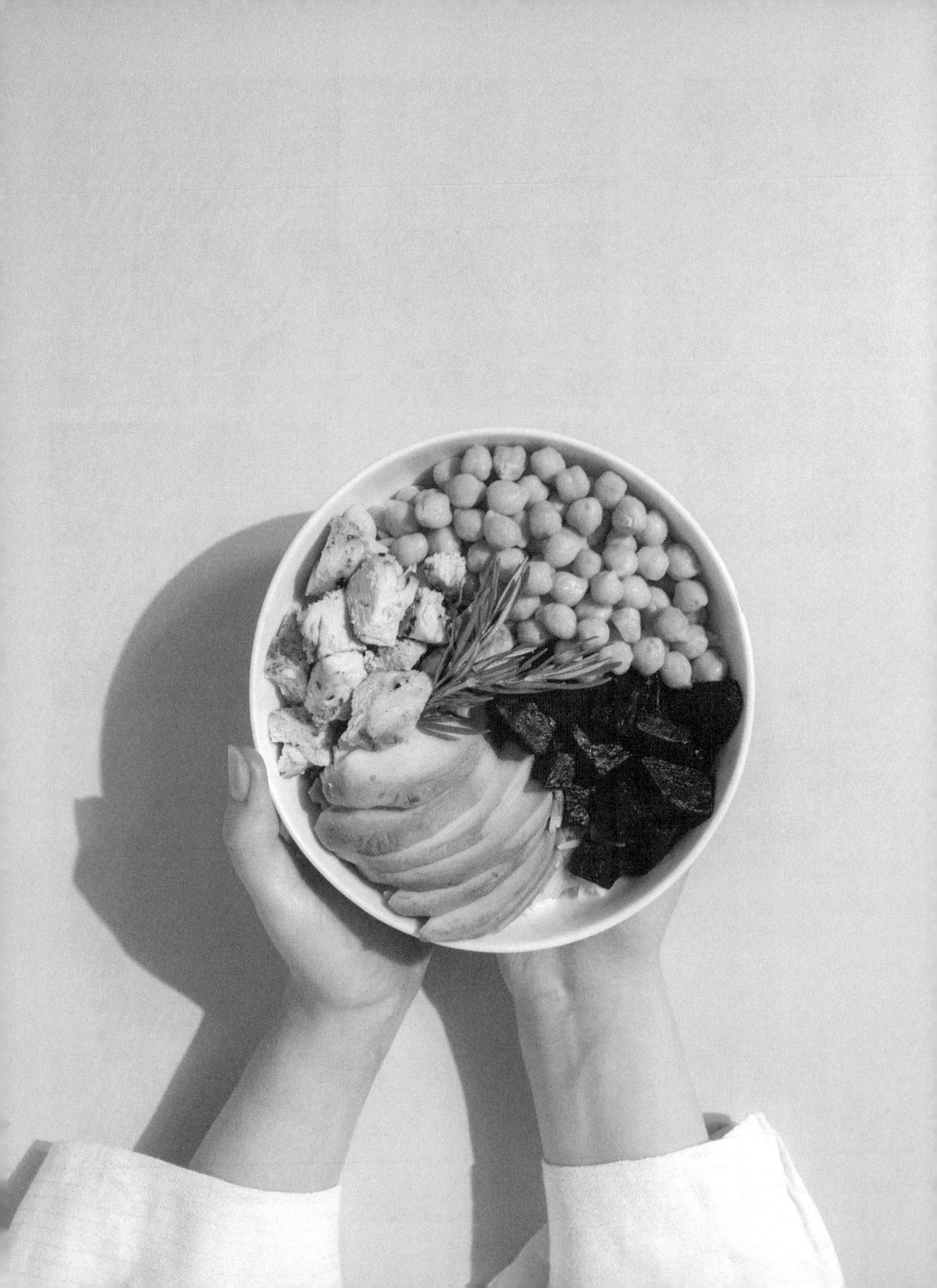

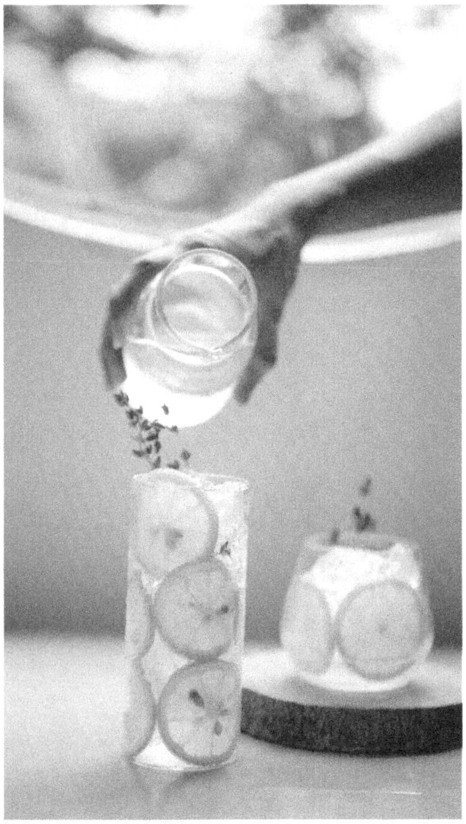
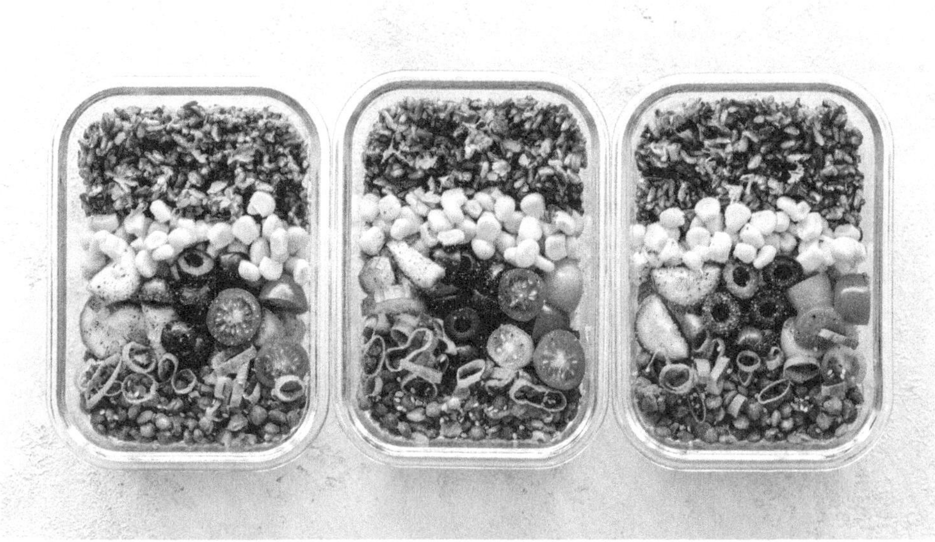
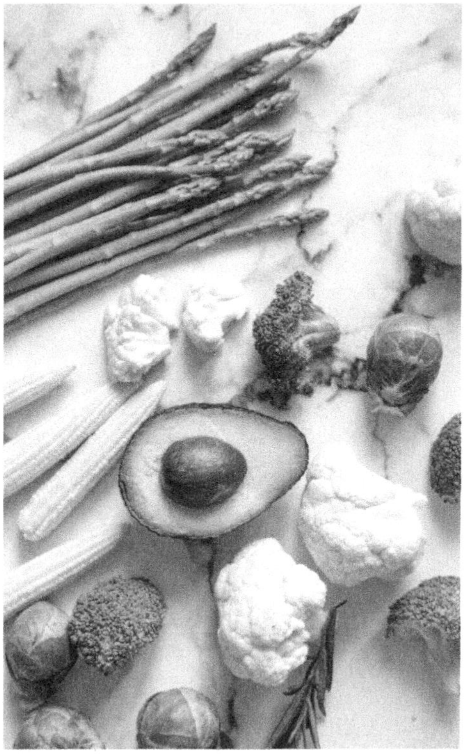
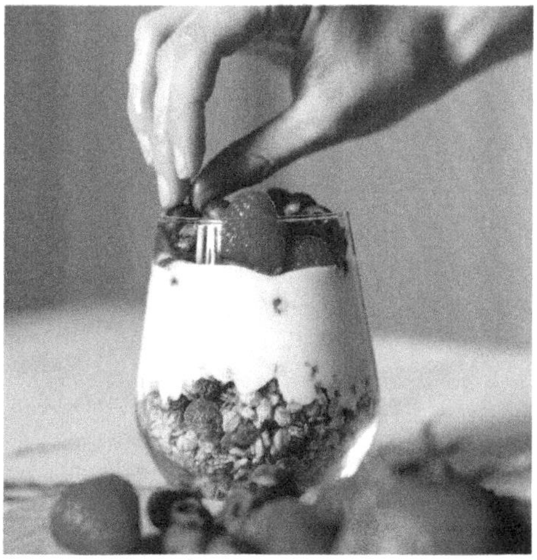
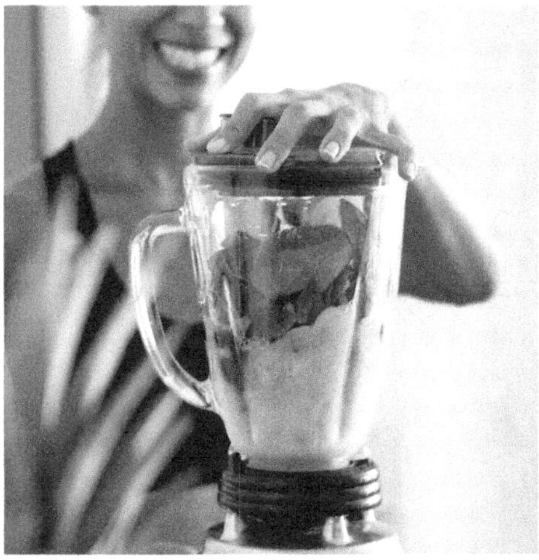
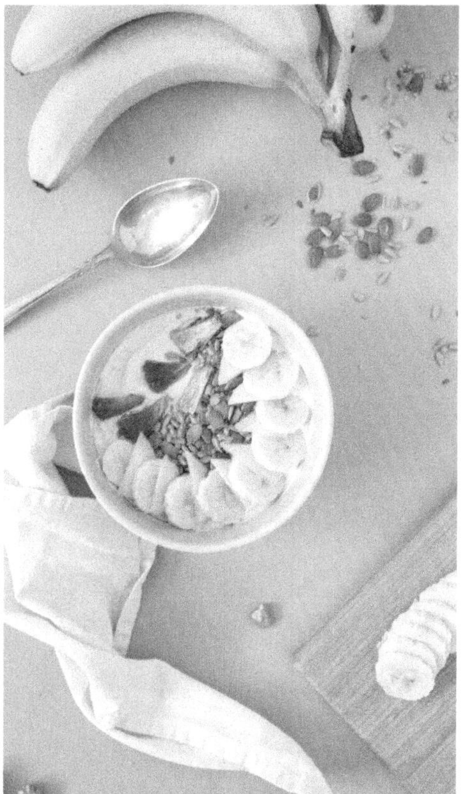
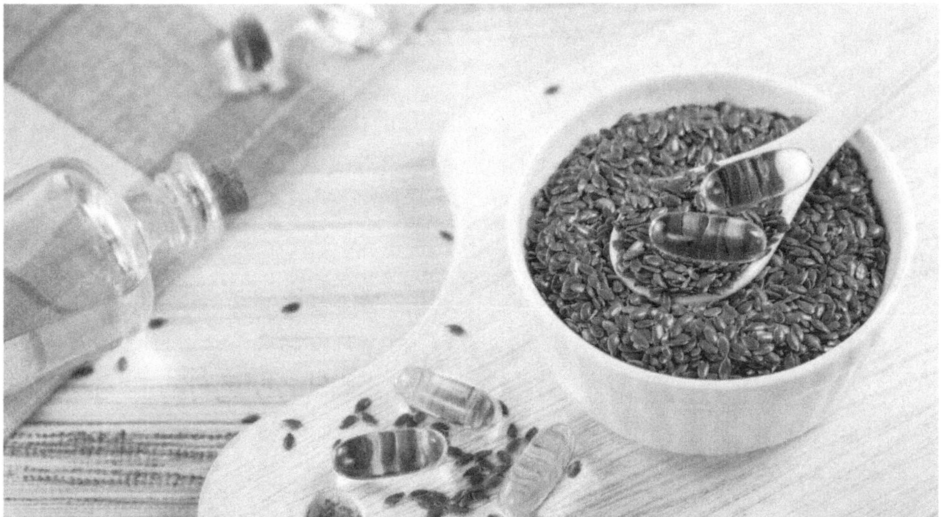

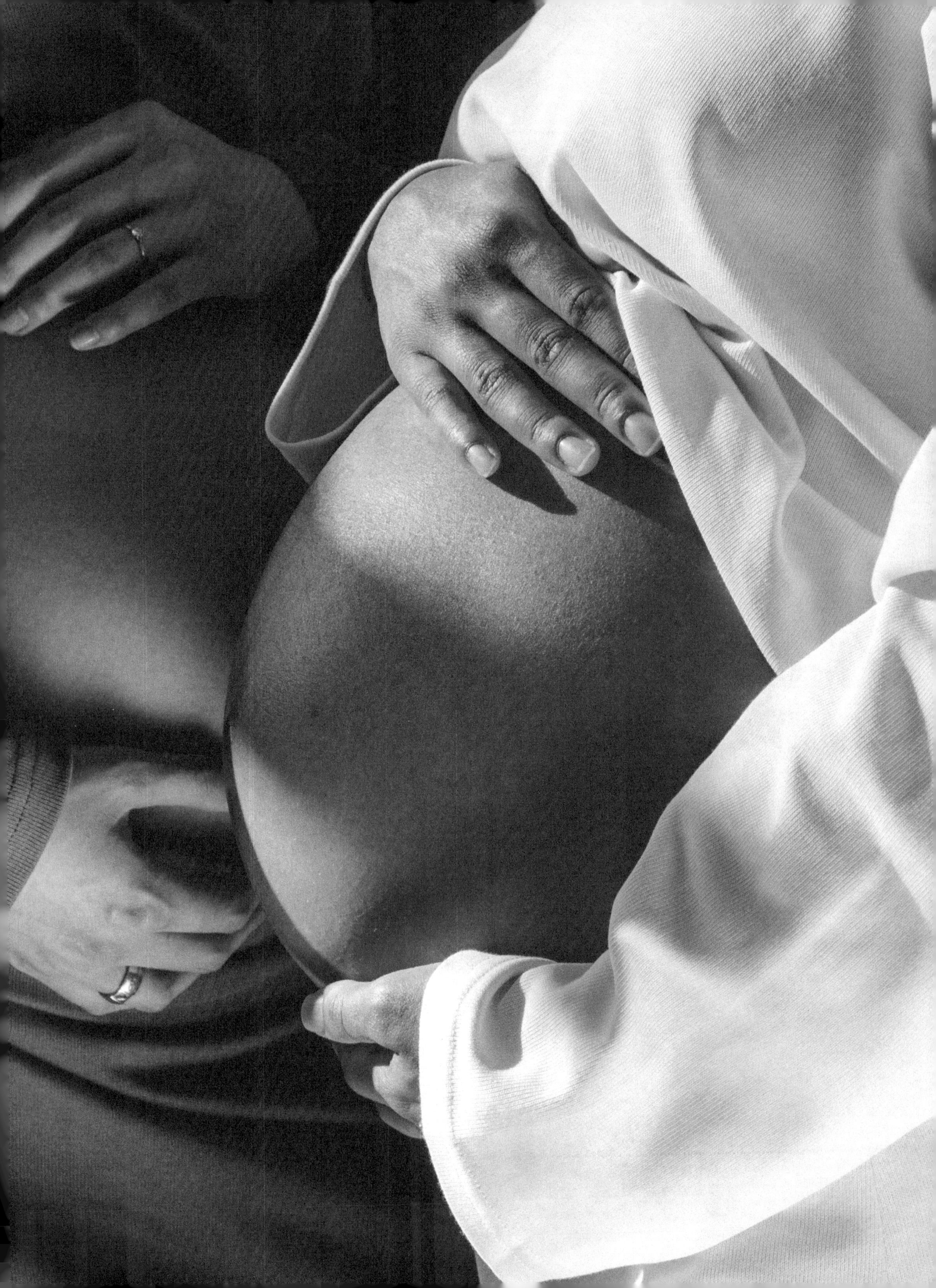

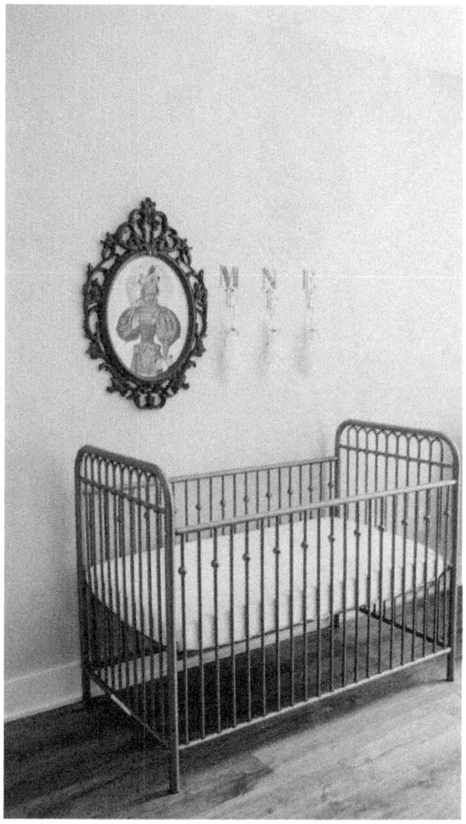
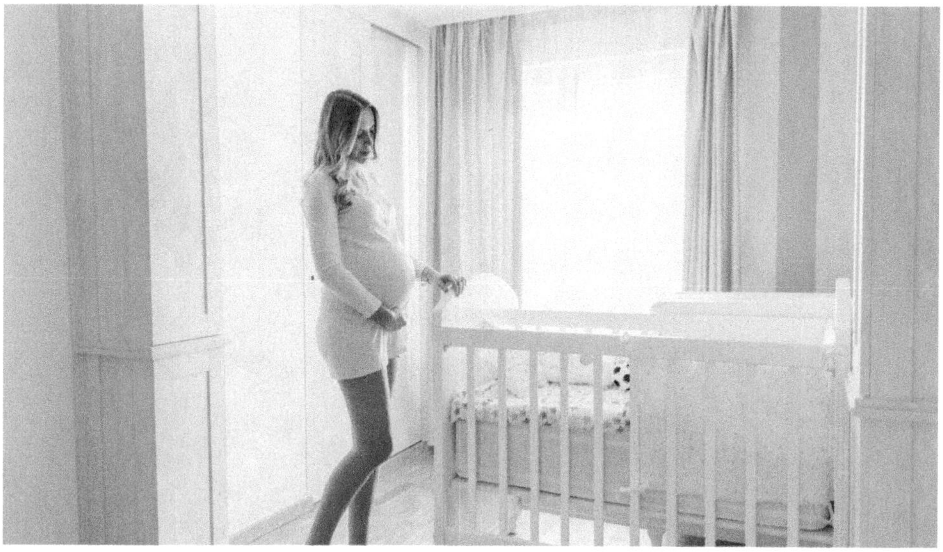
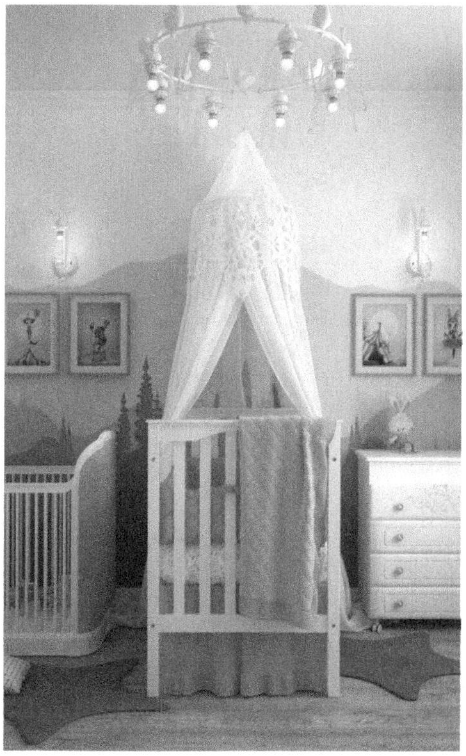
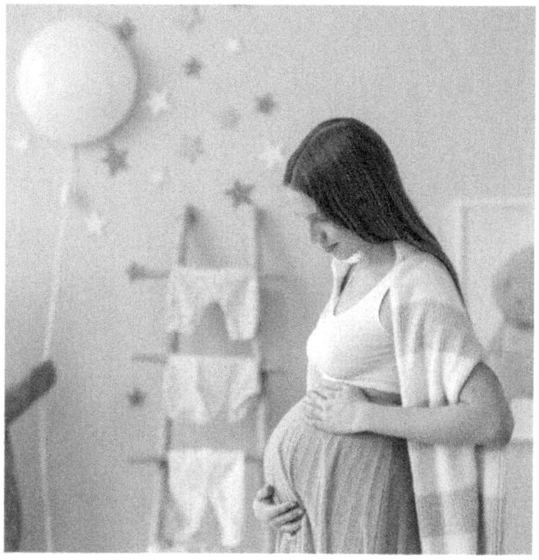
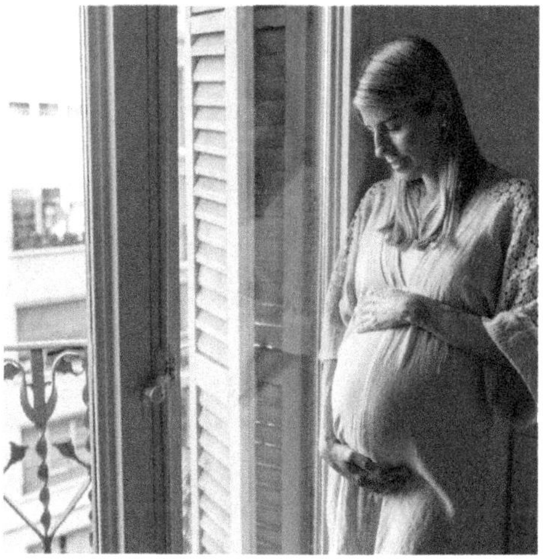
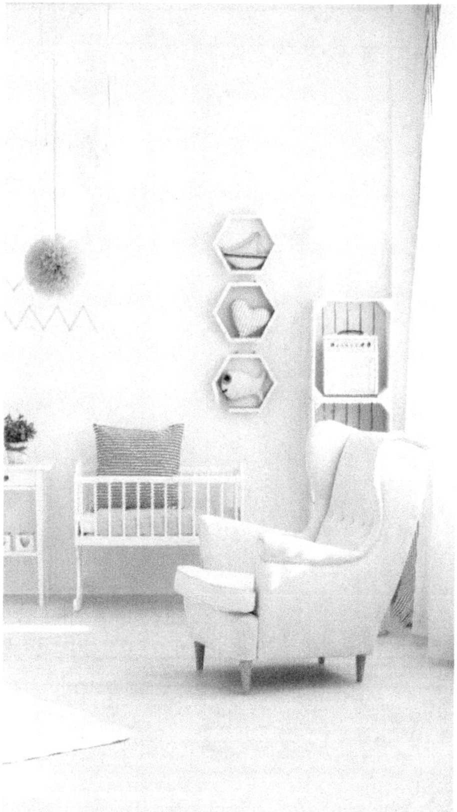
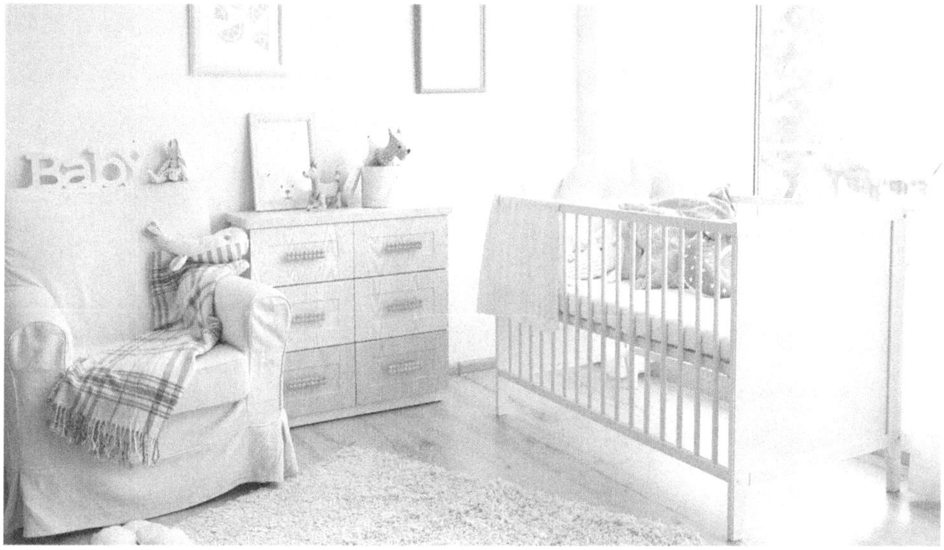
Baby

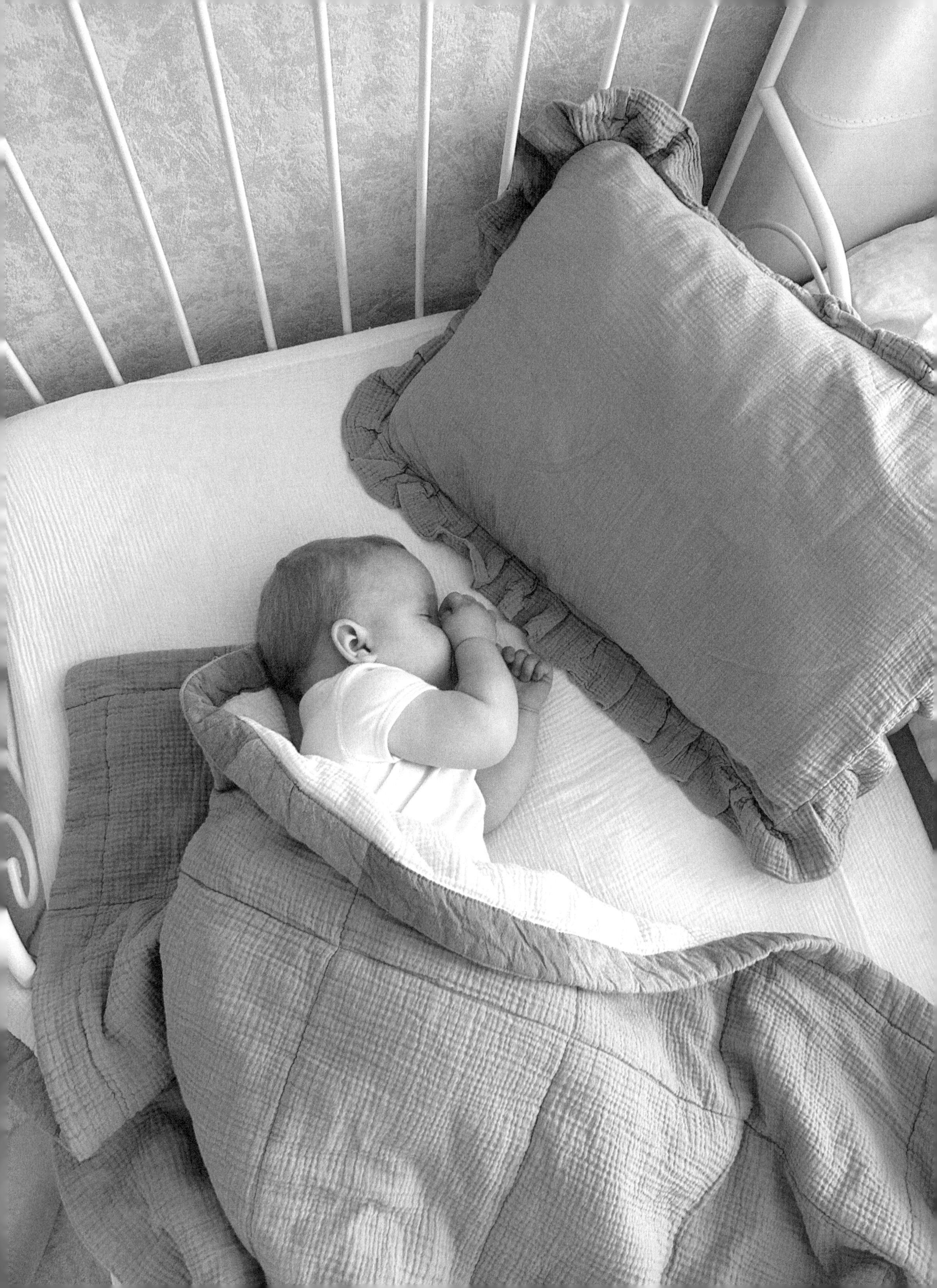

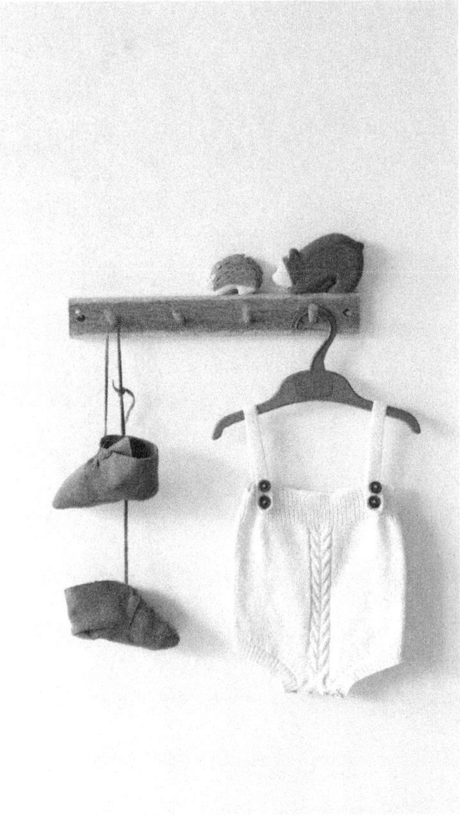
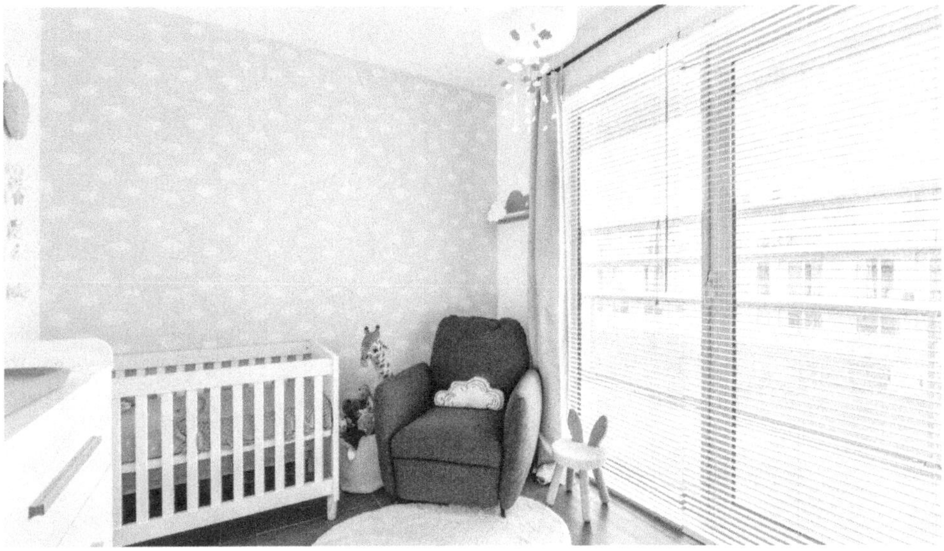
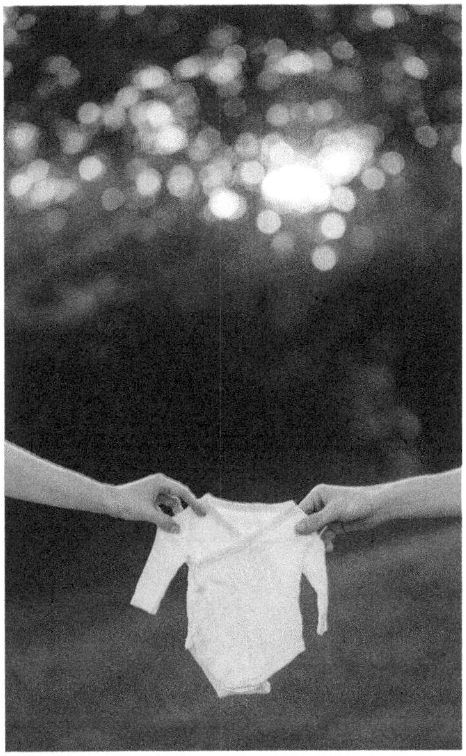
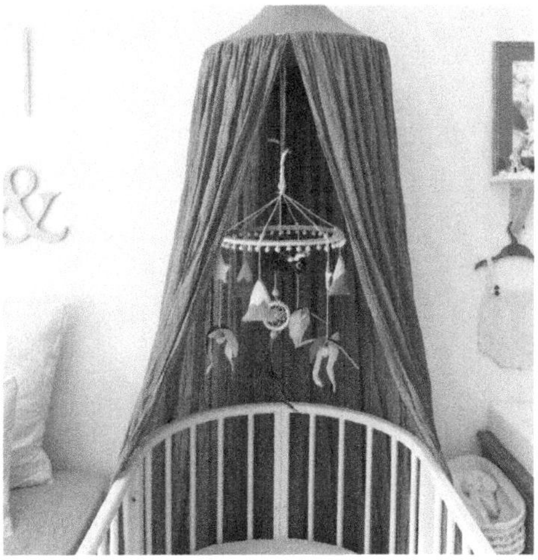
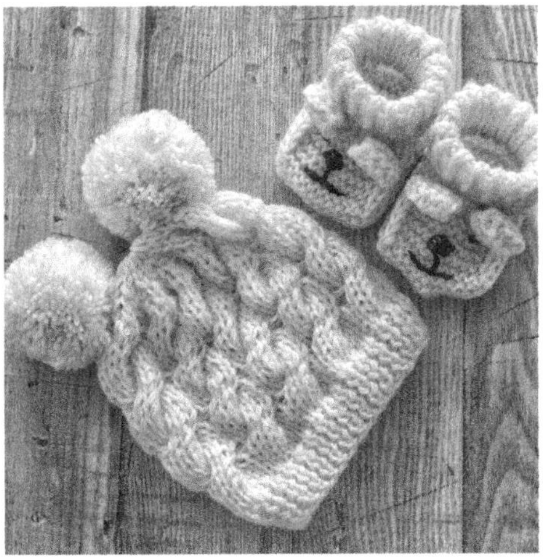
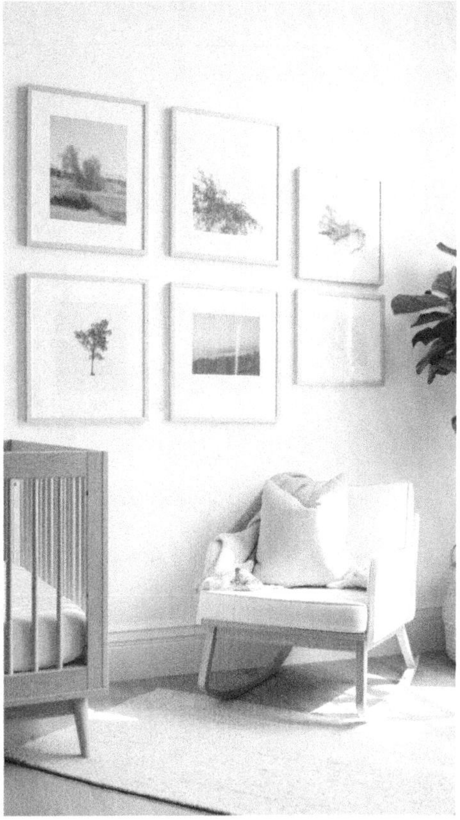
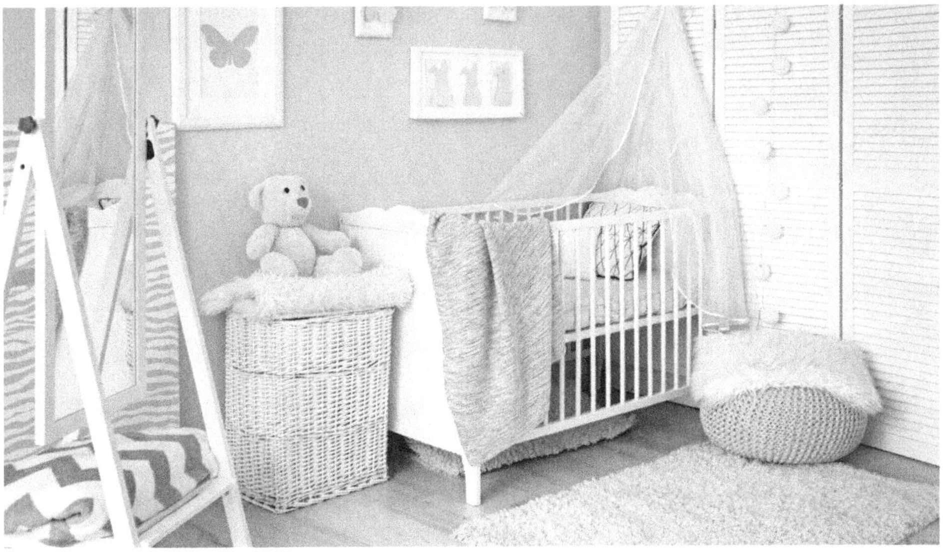

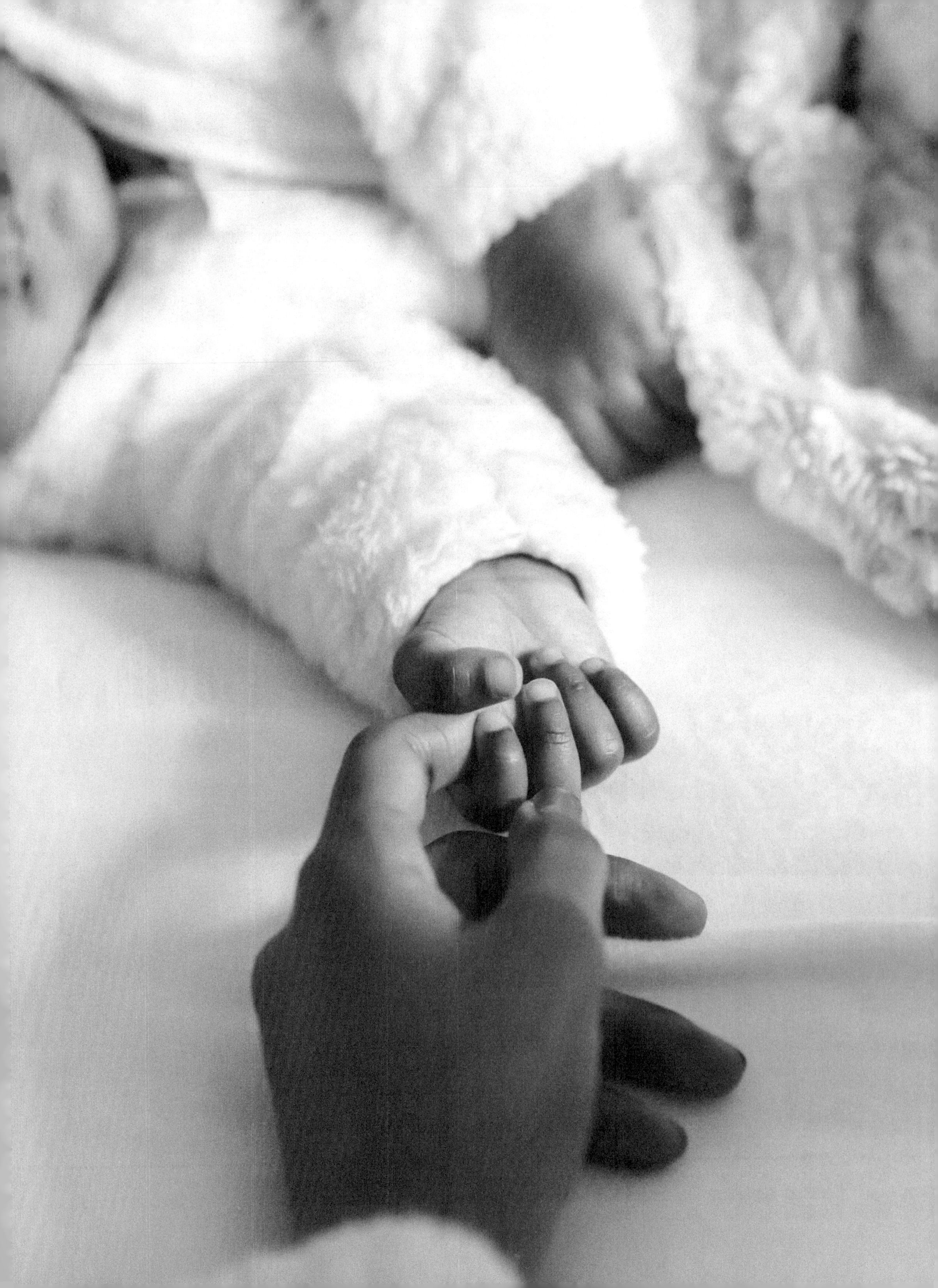

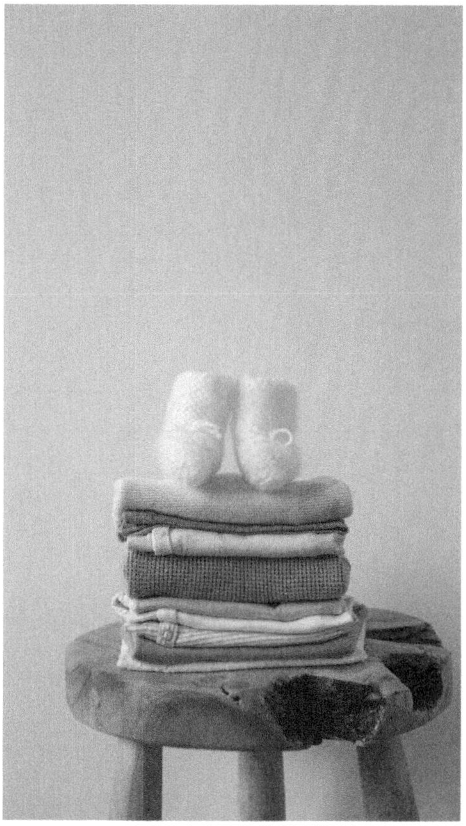
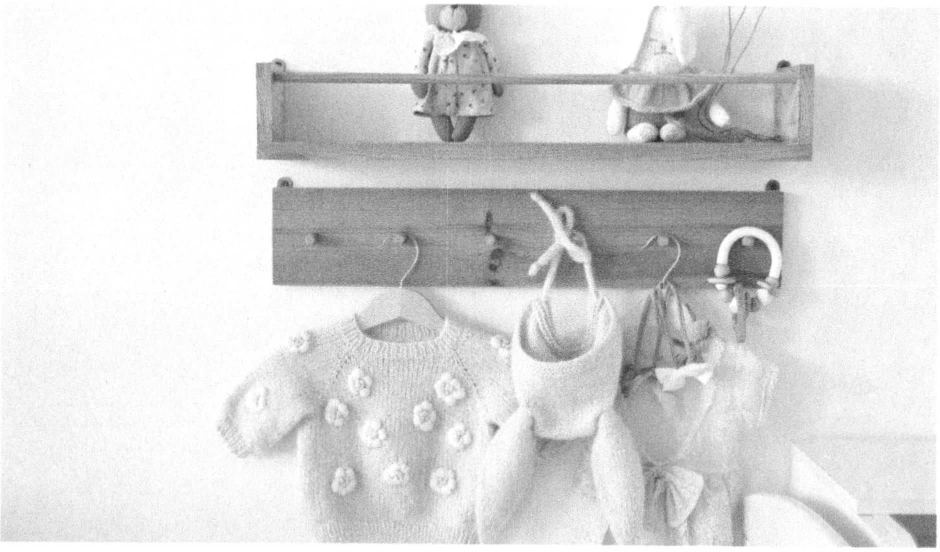
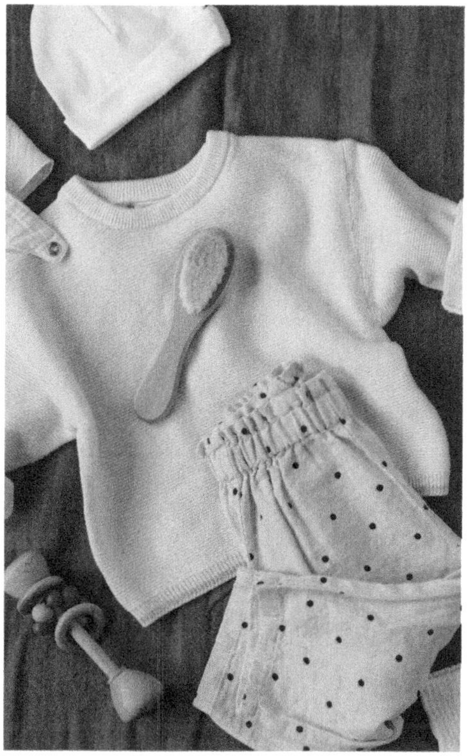
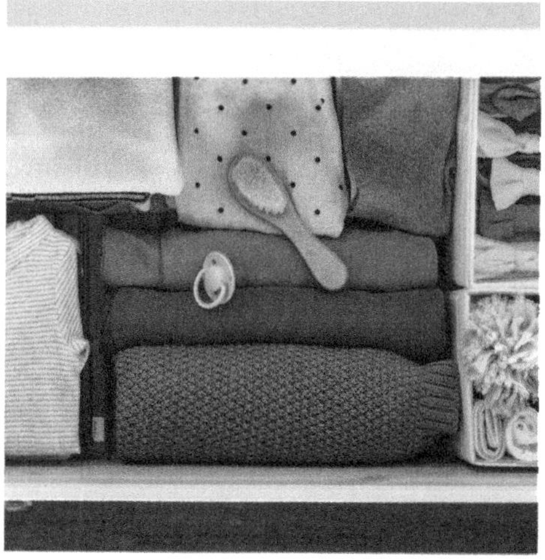
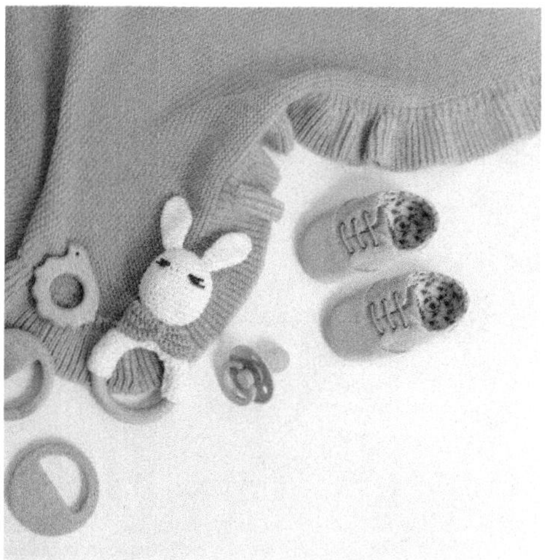
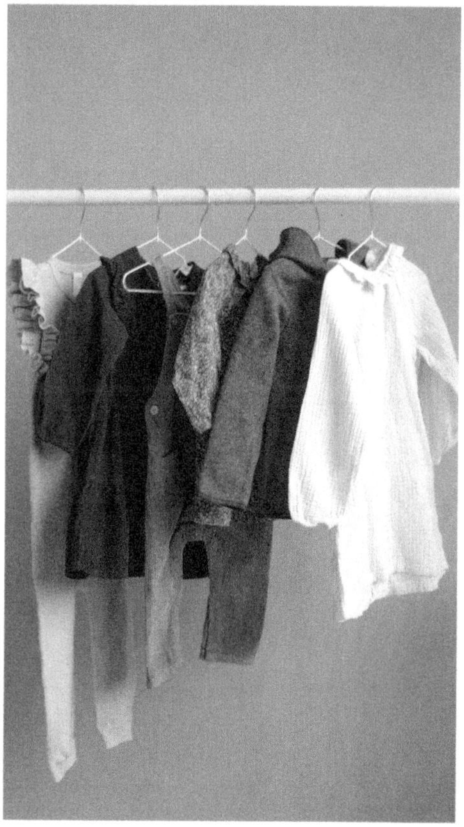
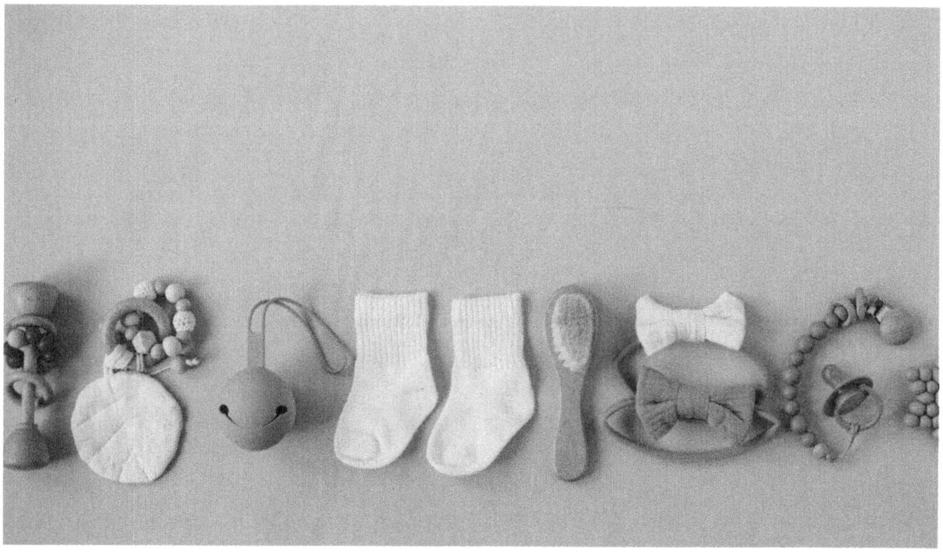

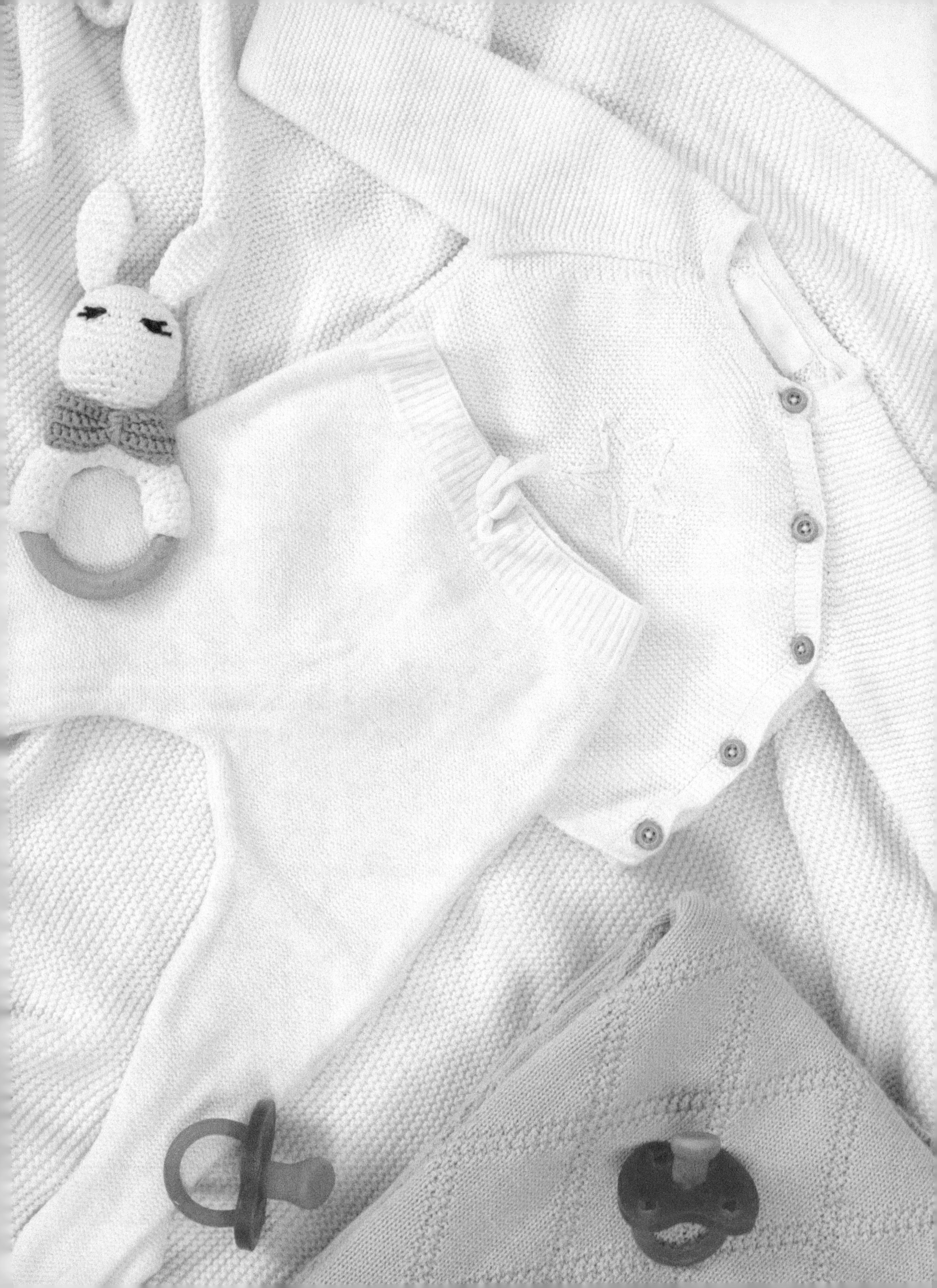

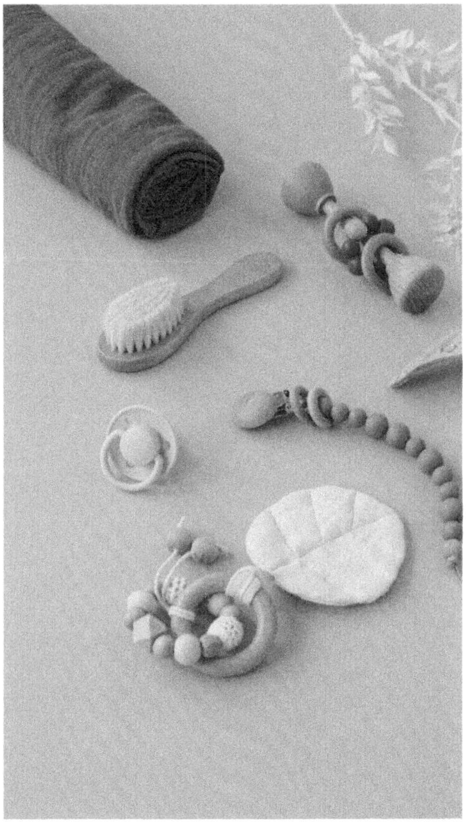
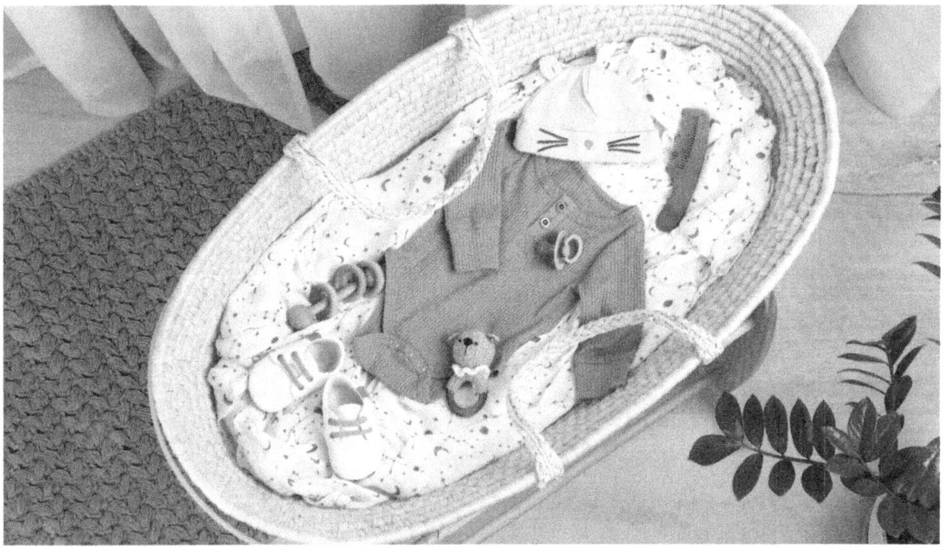
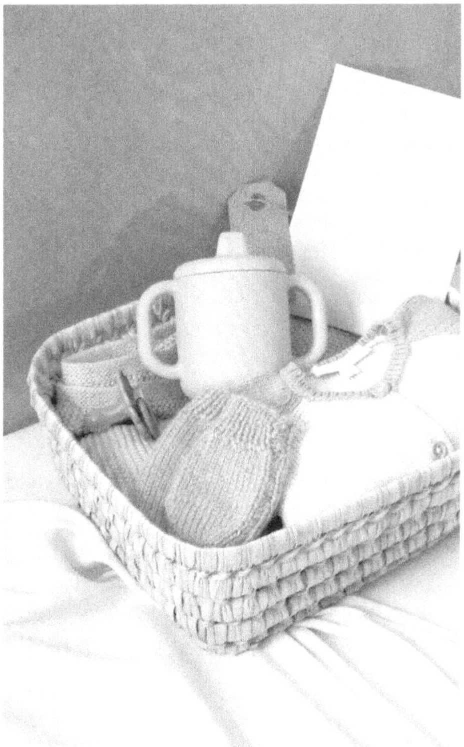
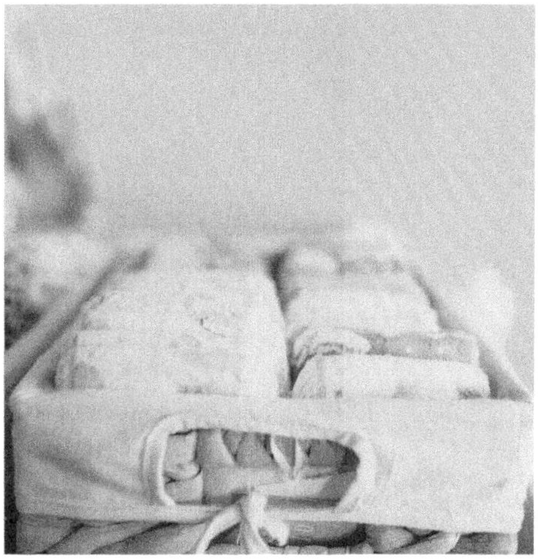
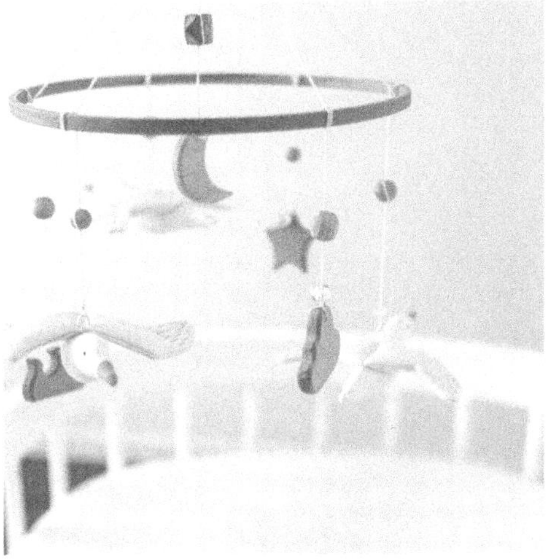
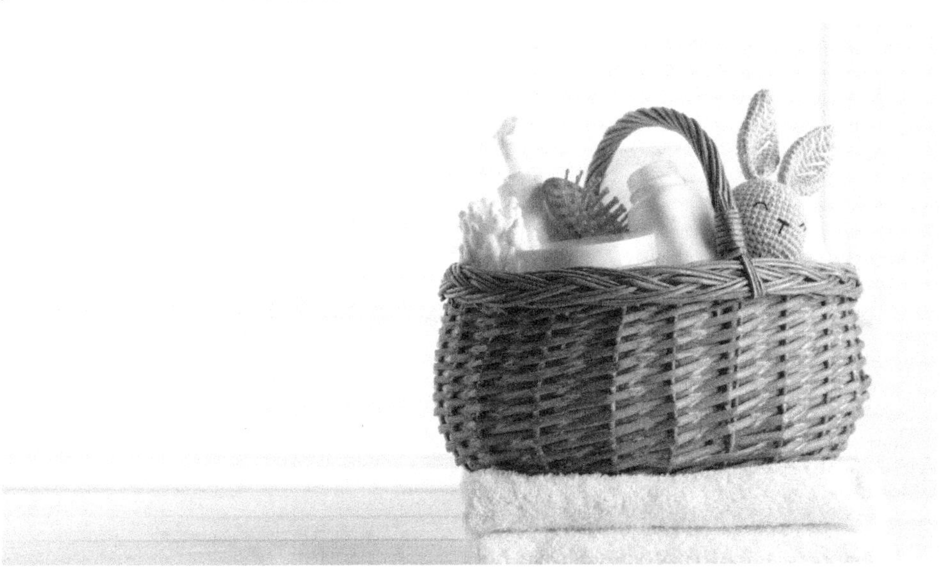
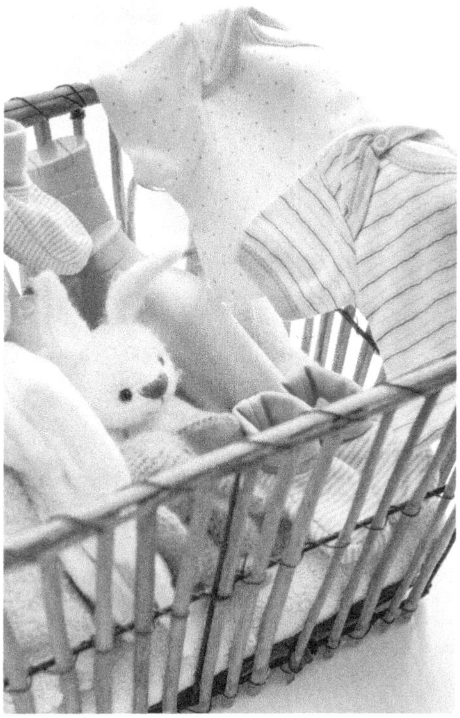

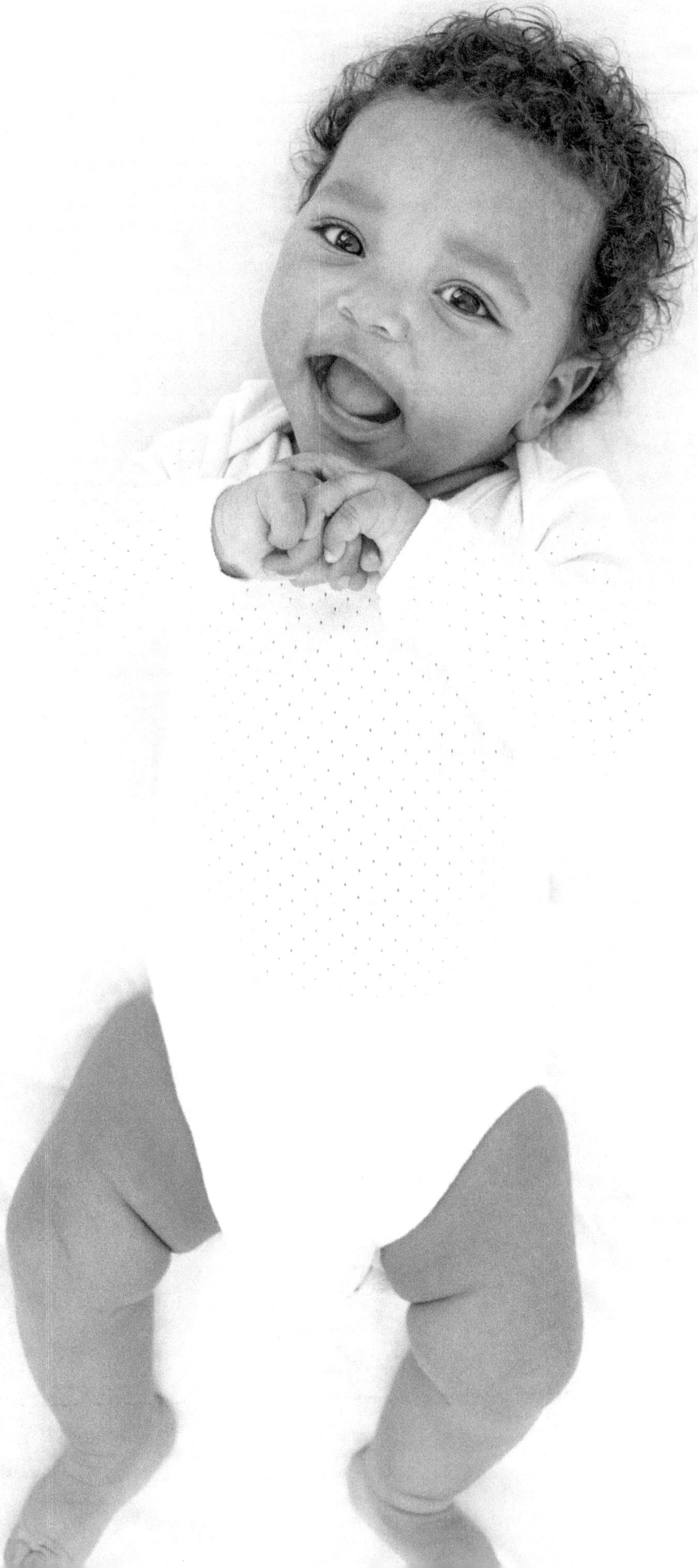

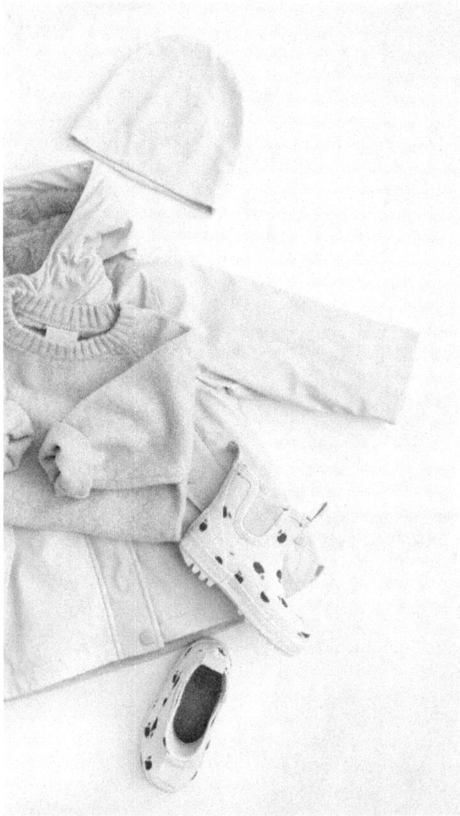

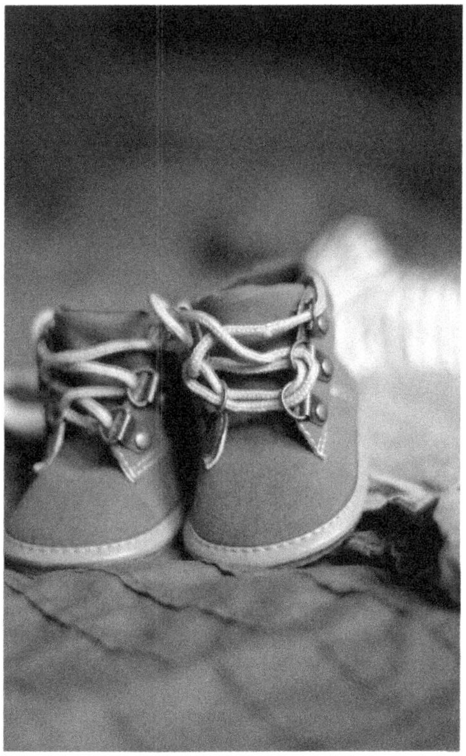
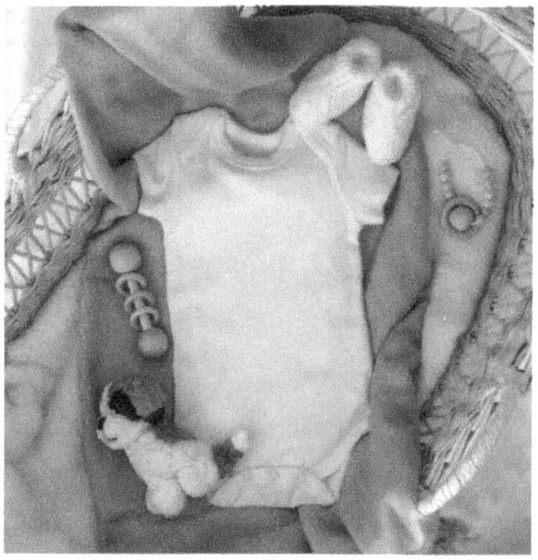
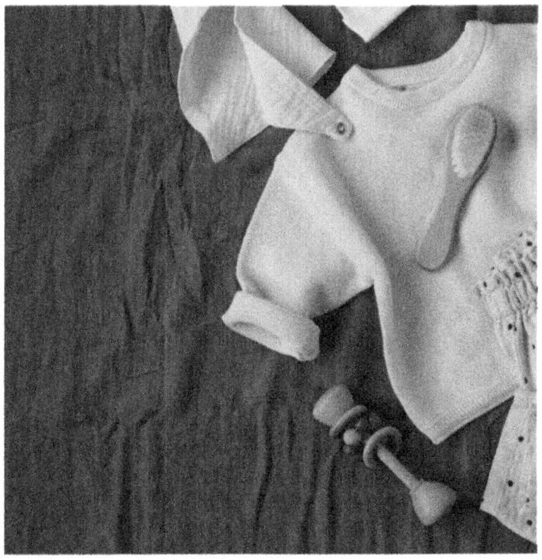
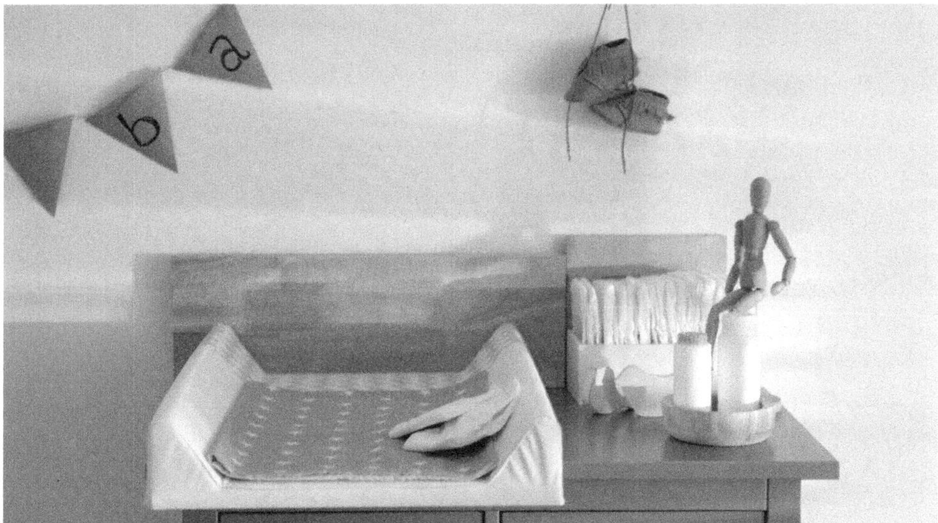
b
a
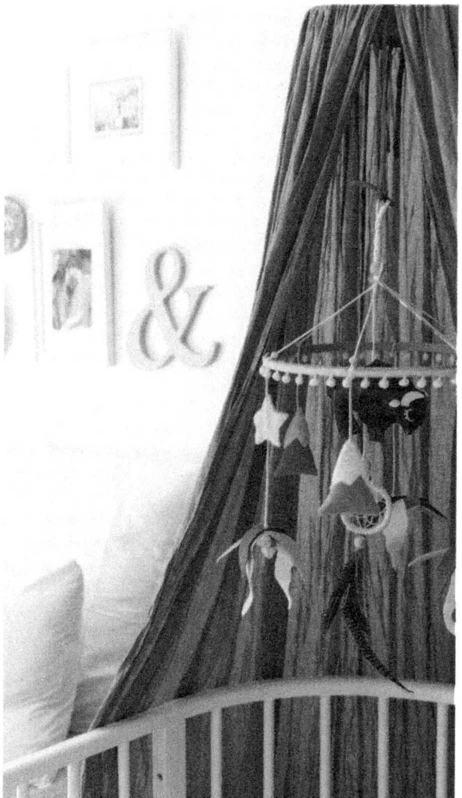
&

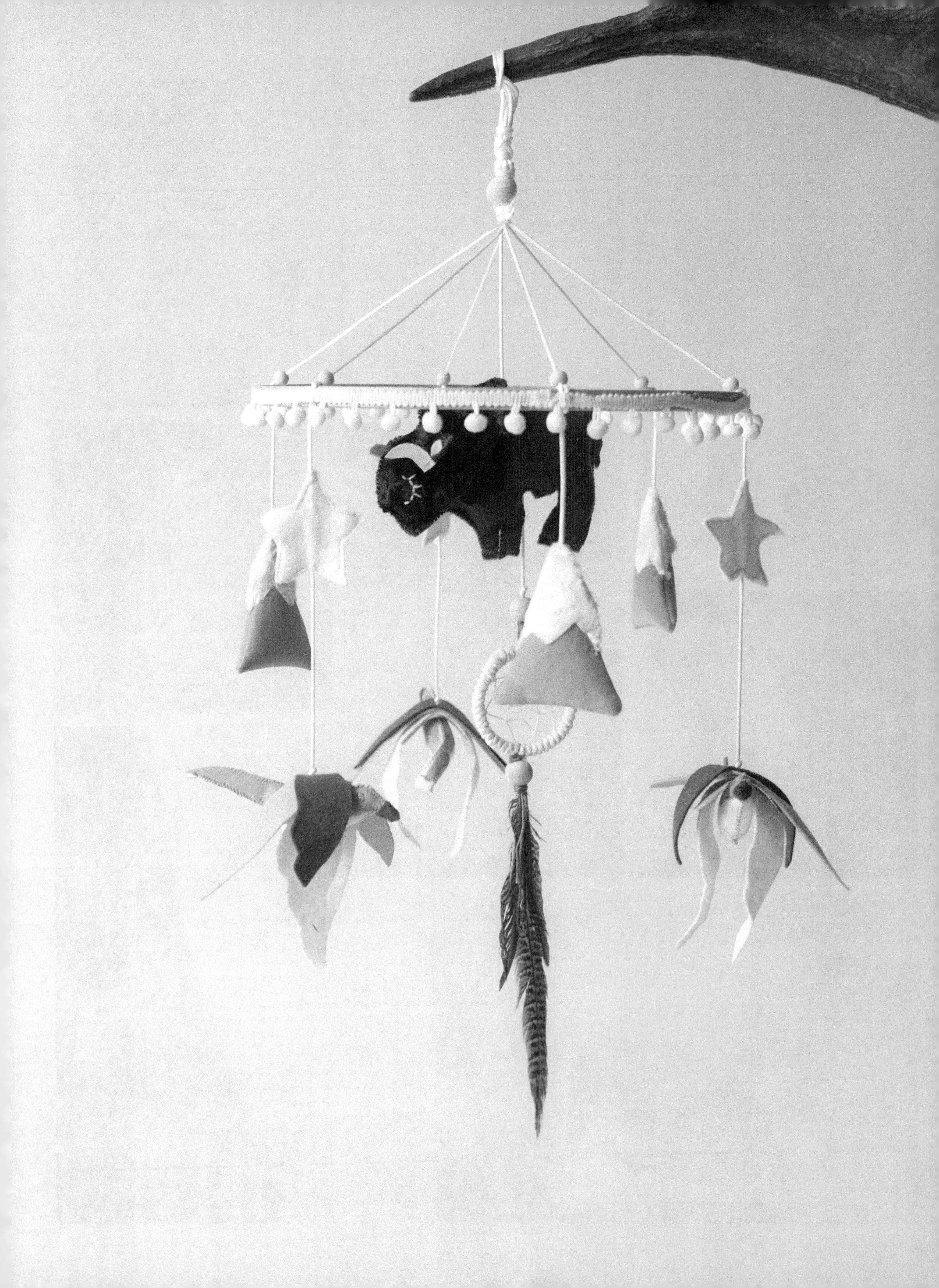

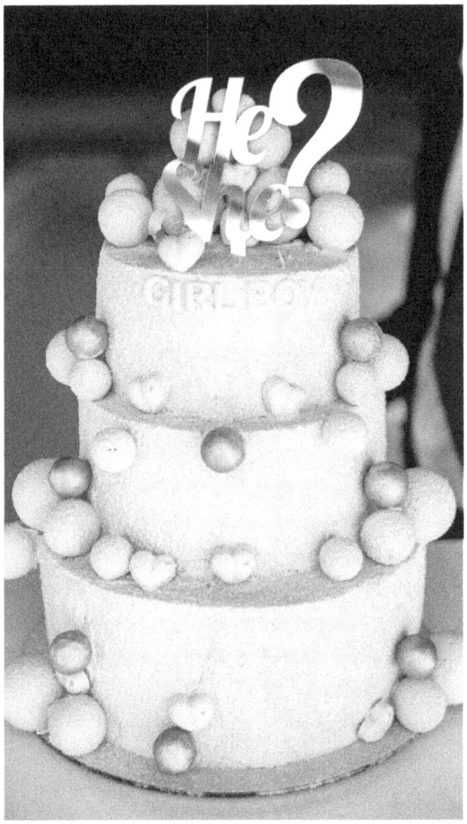
He
?
GIRL BOY

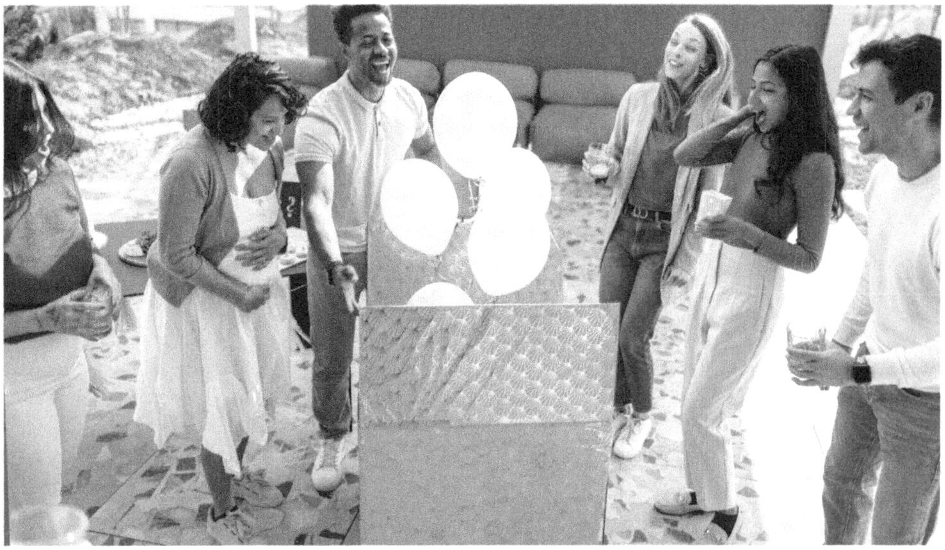

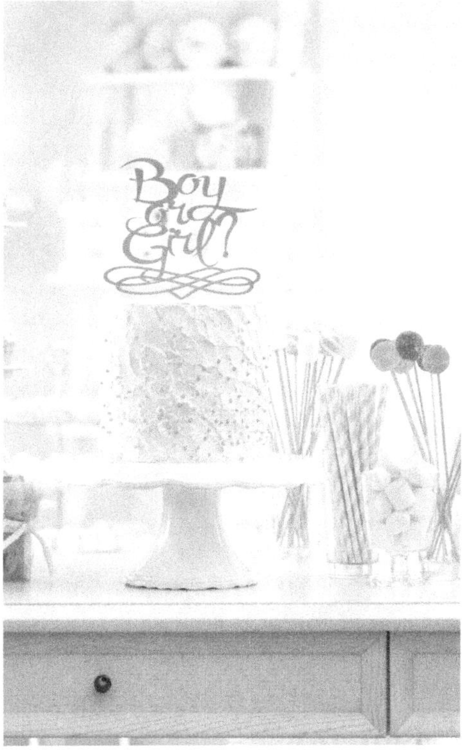
Boy or Girl?

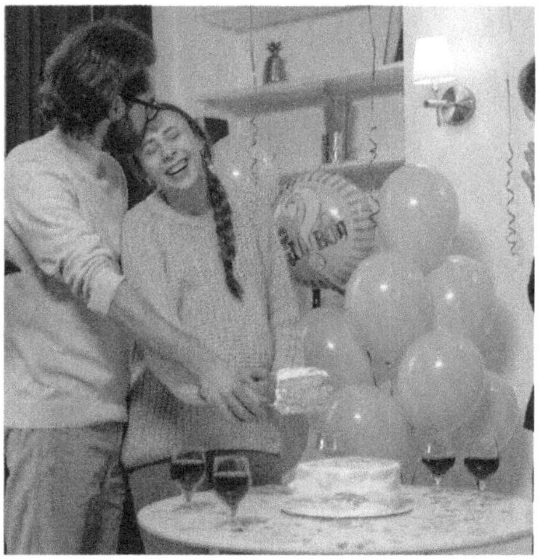

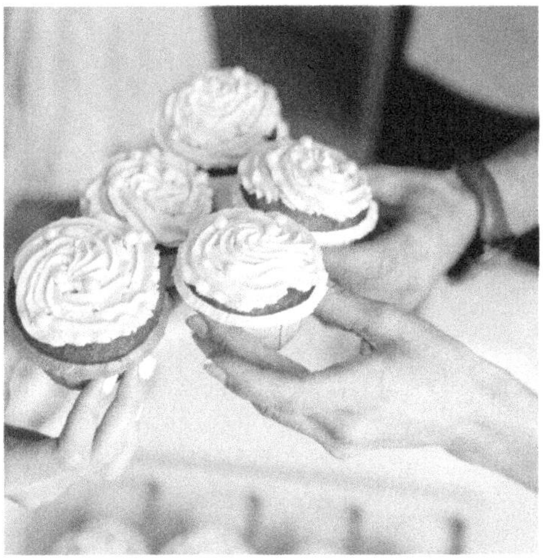

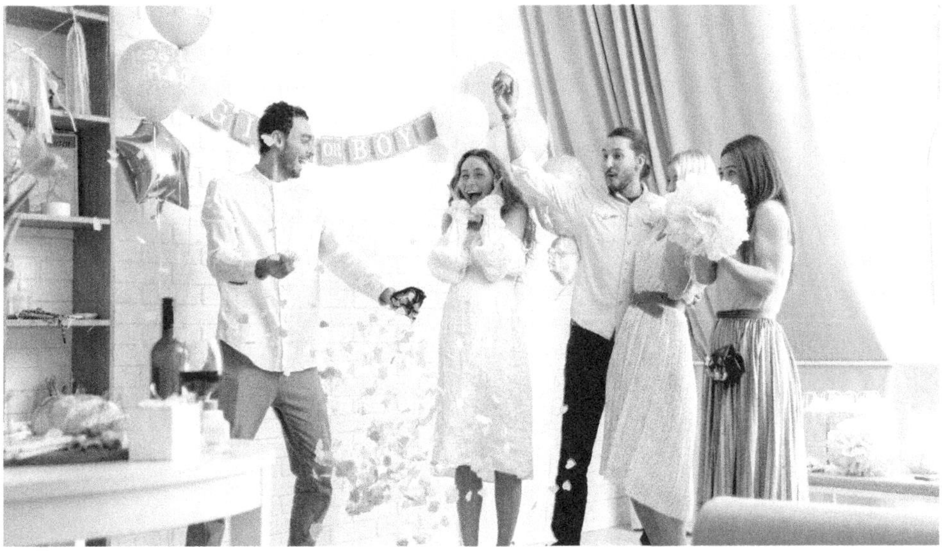

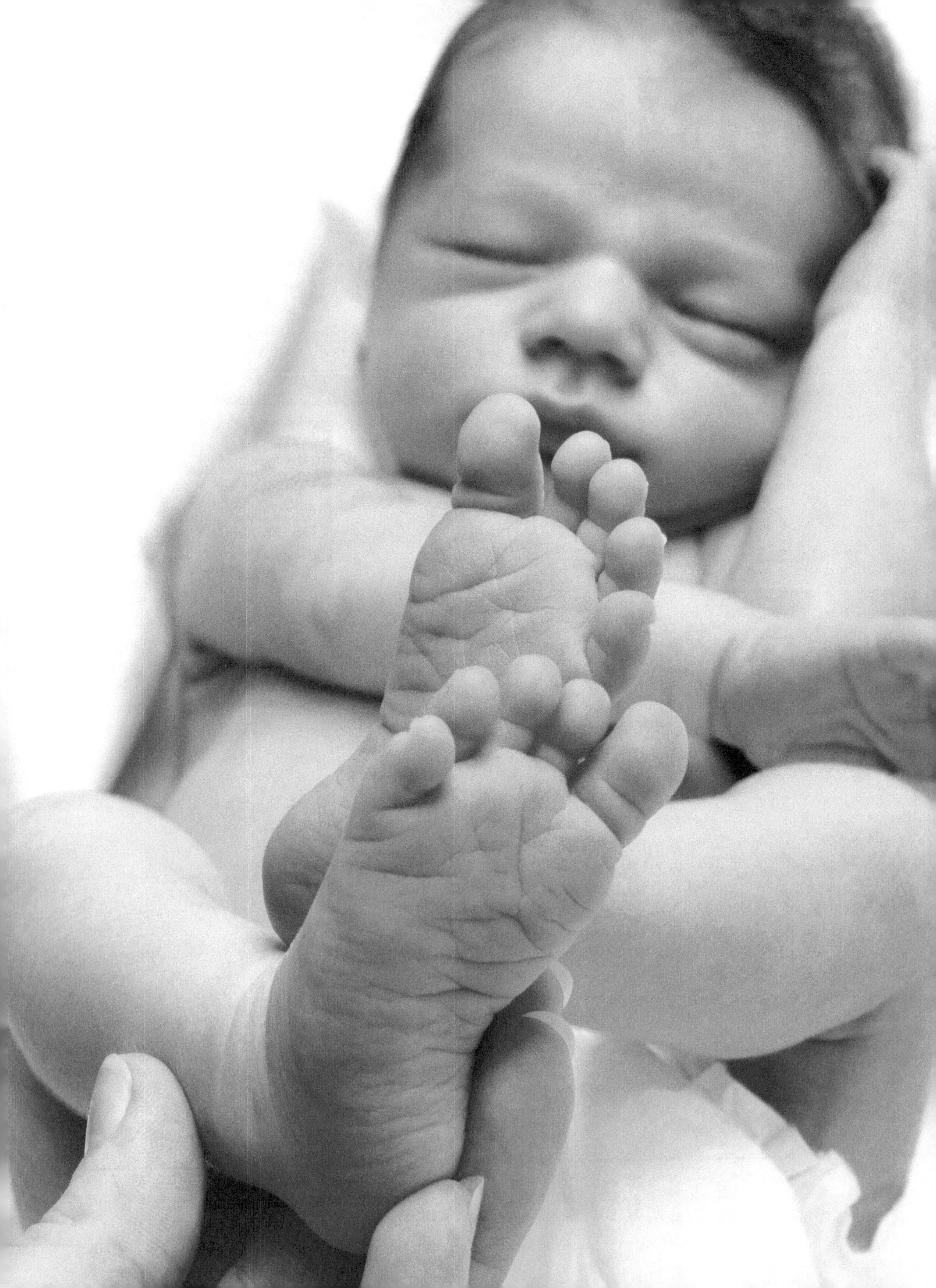

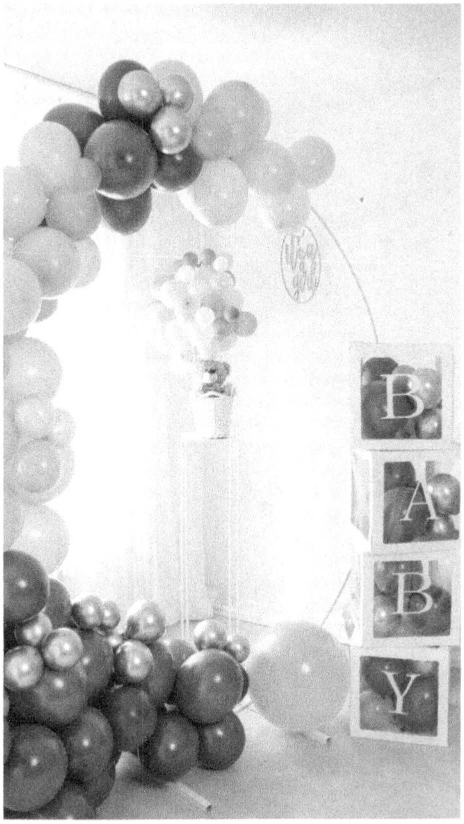
B
A
B
Y
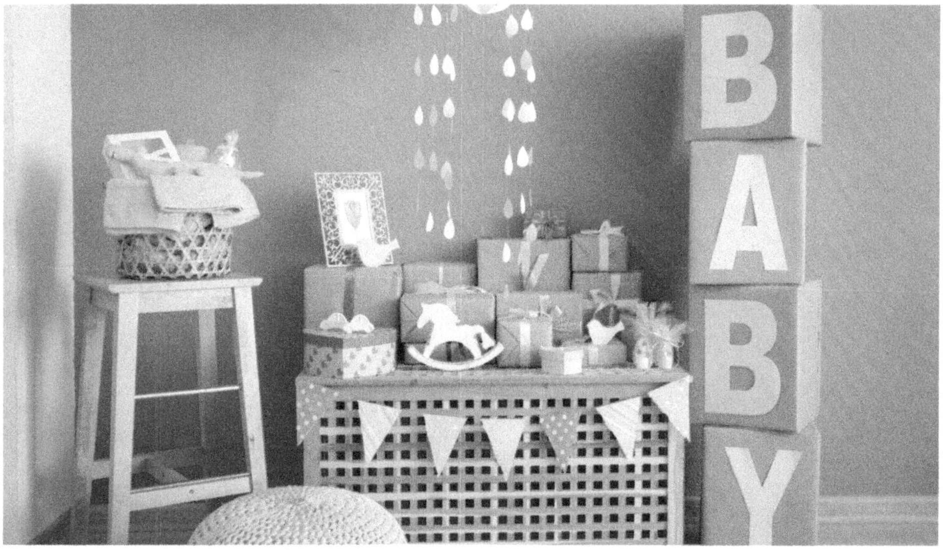
B
A
B
Y
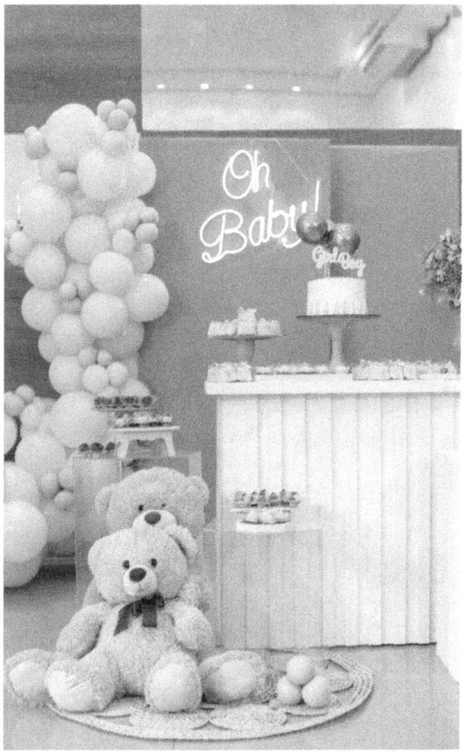
Oh Baby!
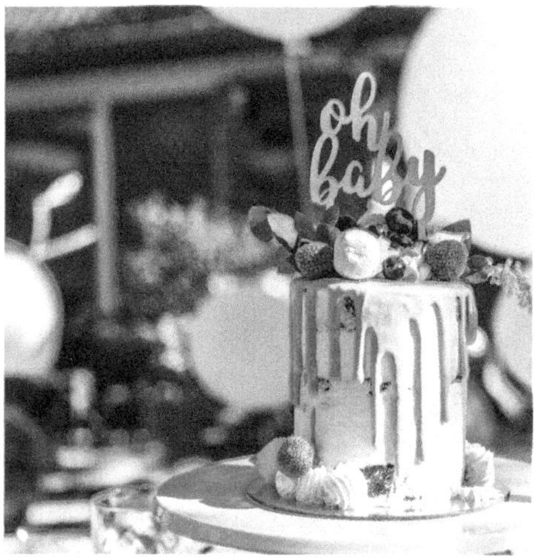
oh baby
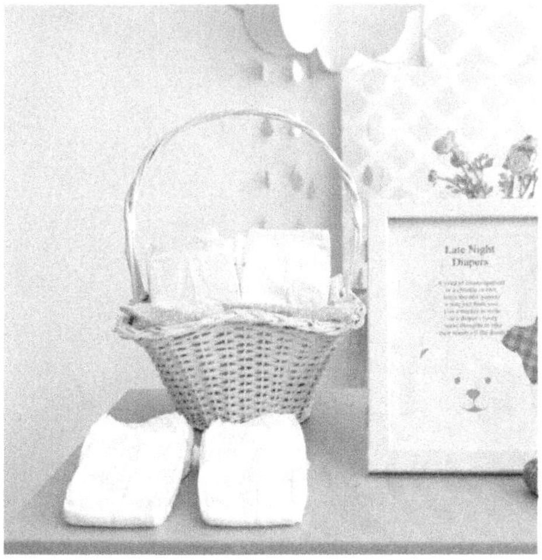
Late Night
Diapers
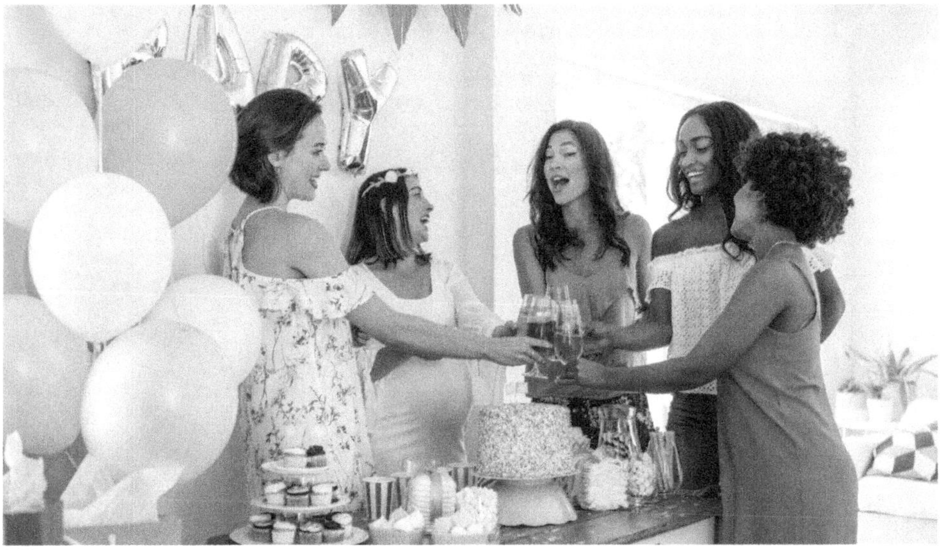
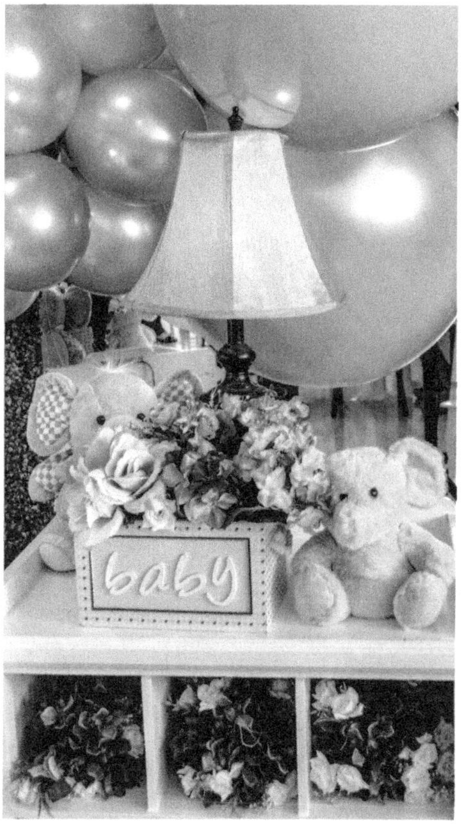
baby

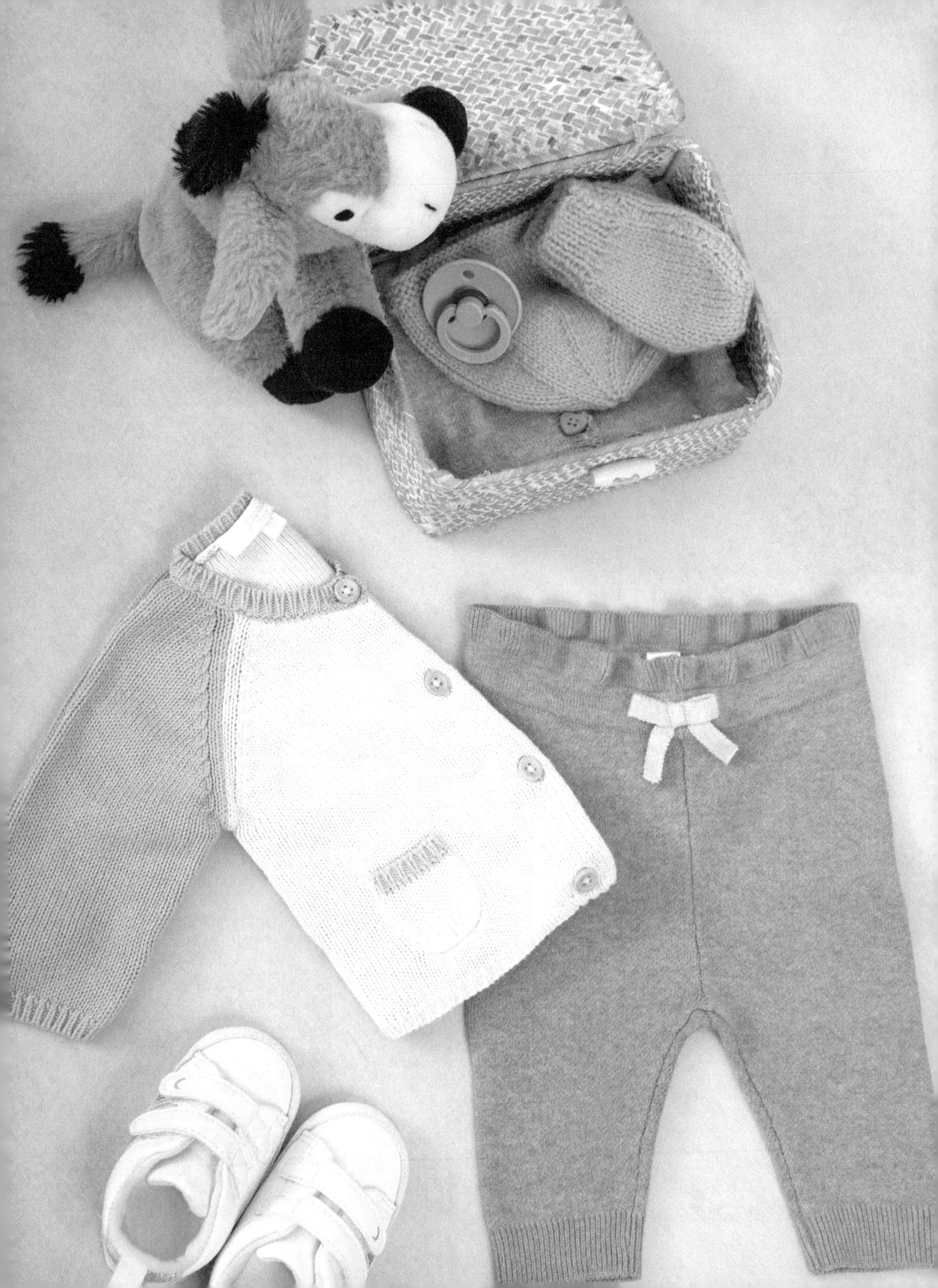

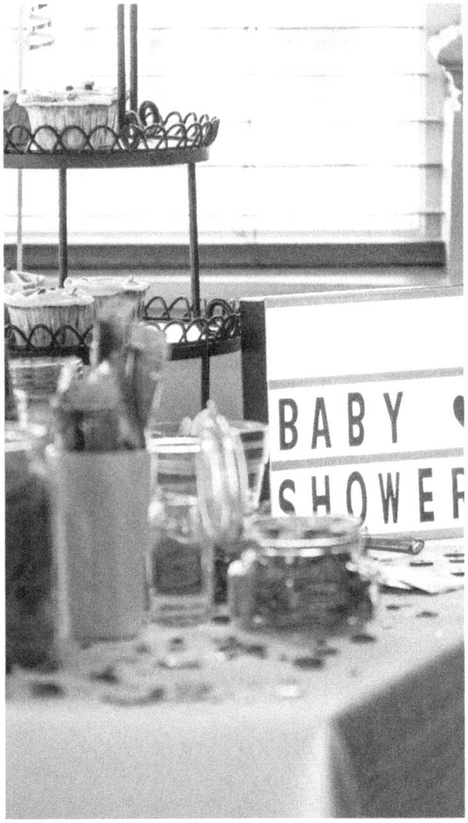
BABY
SHOWER

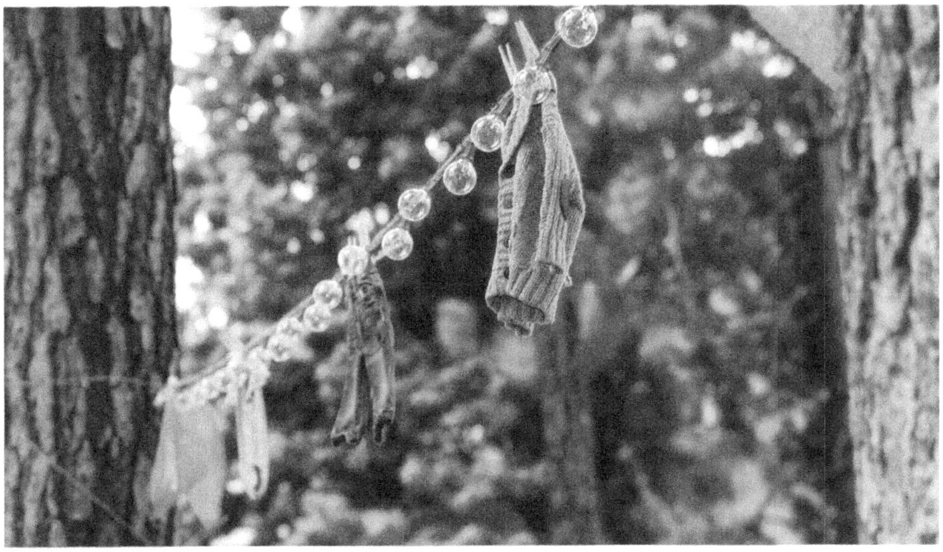

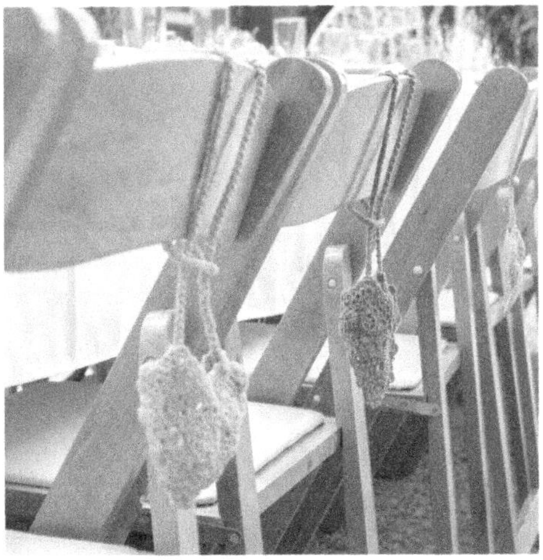

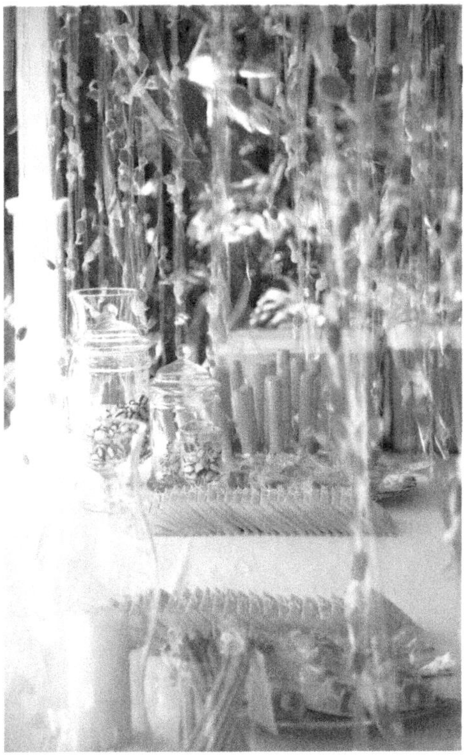

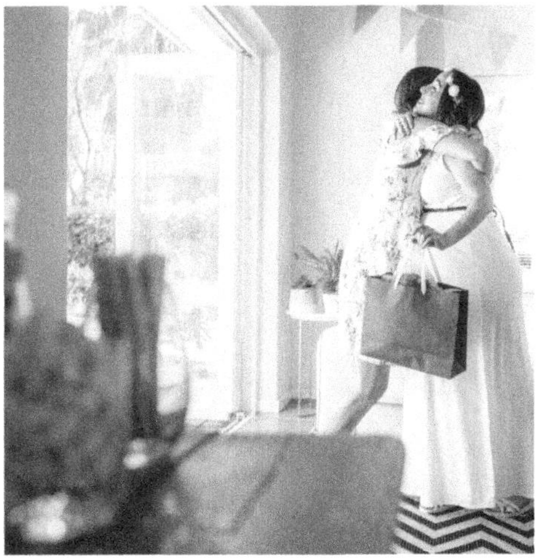

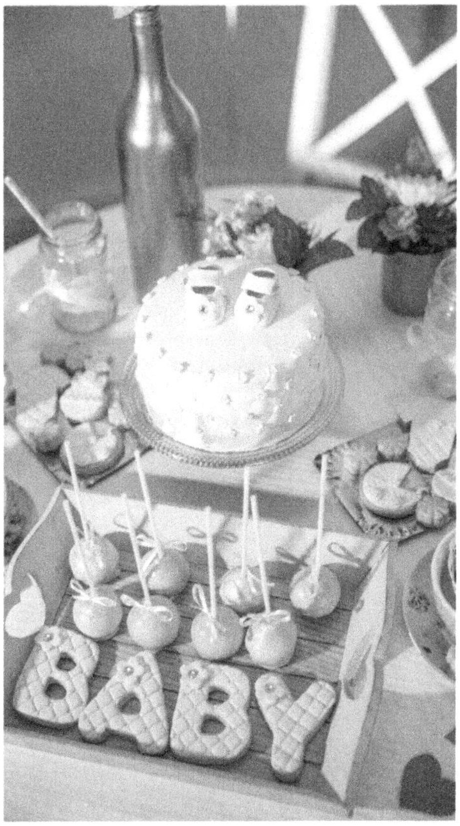
BABY

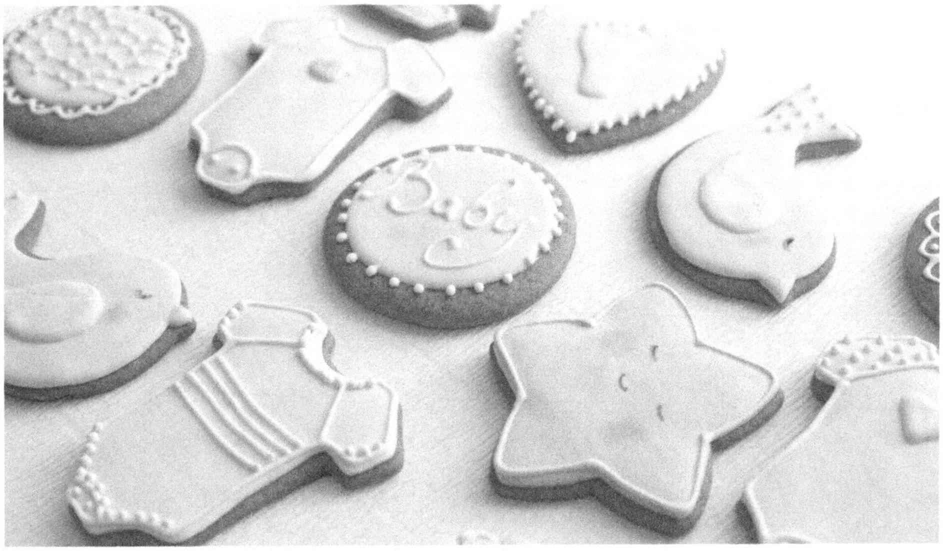
Baby

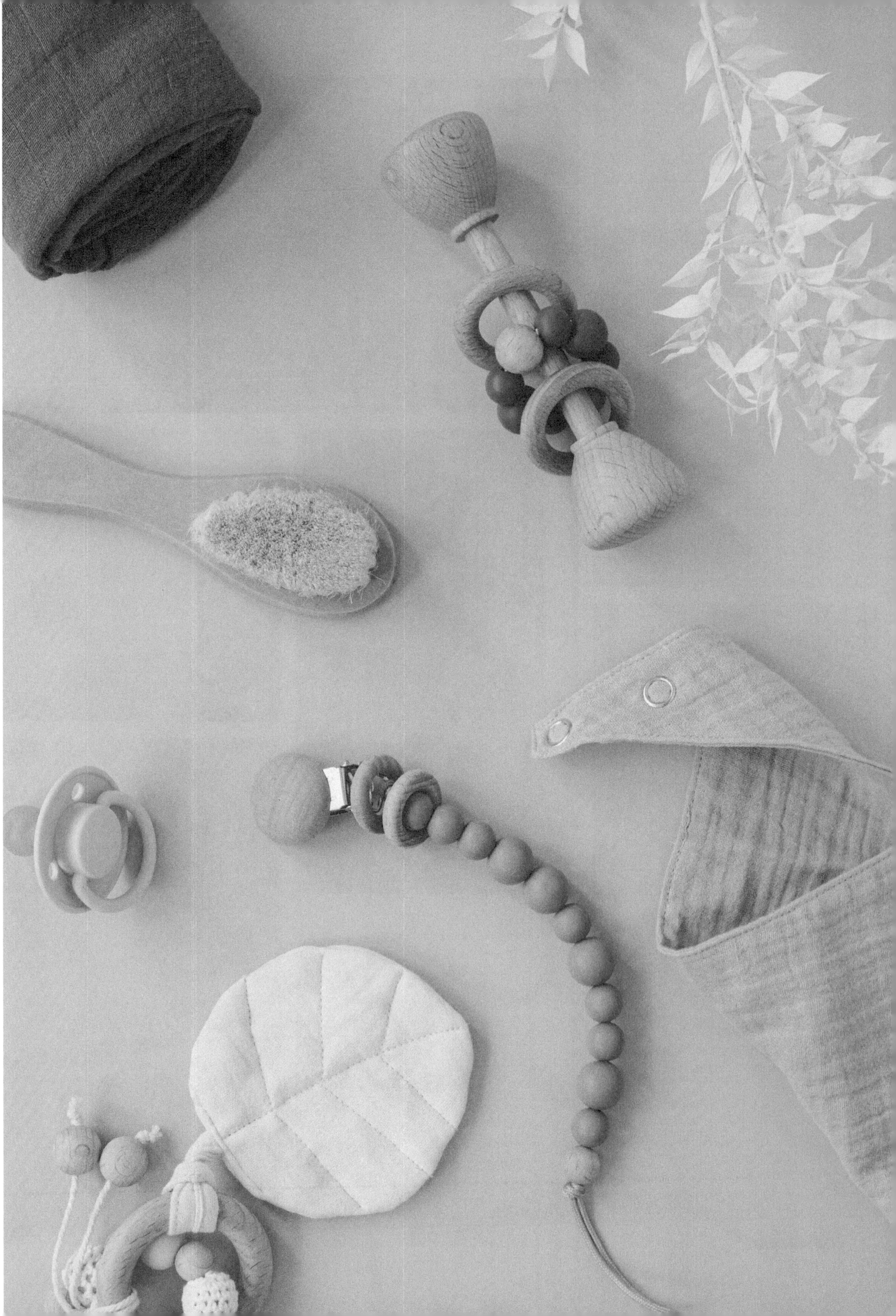

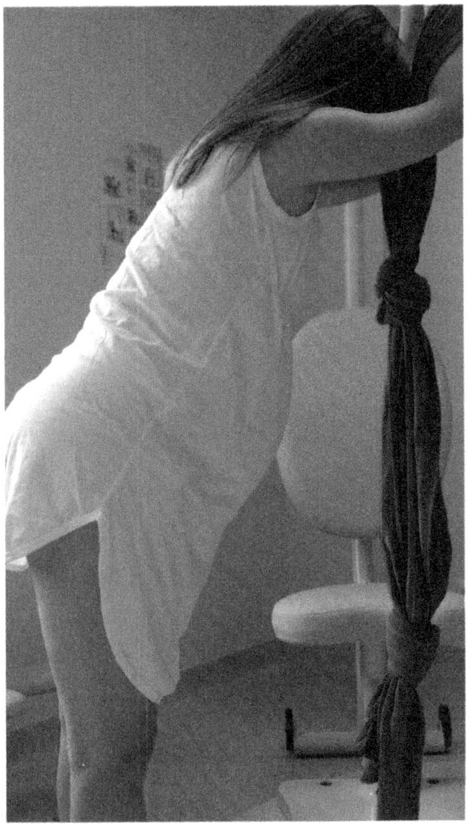

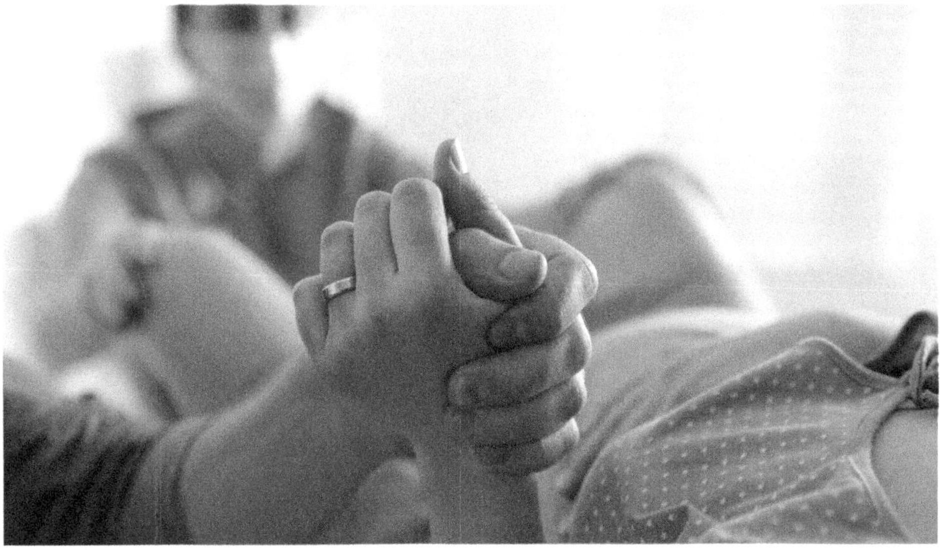

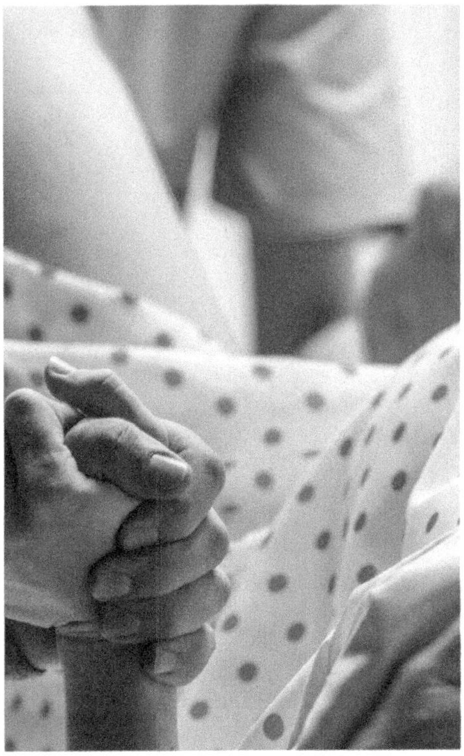

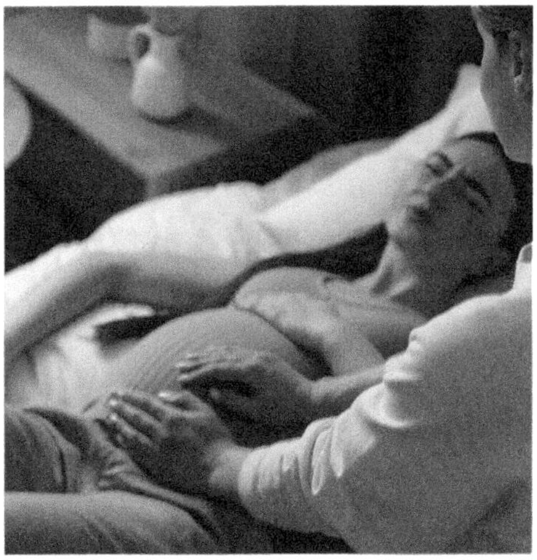

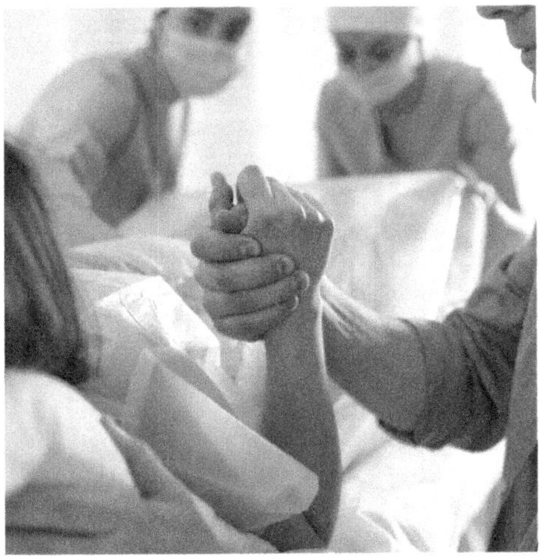

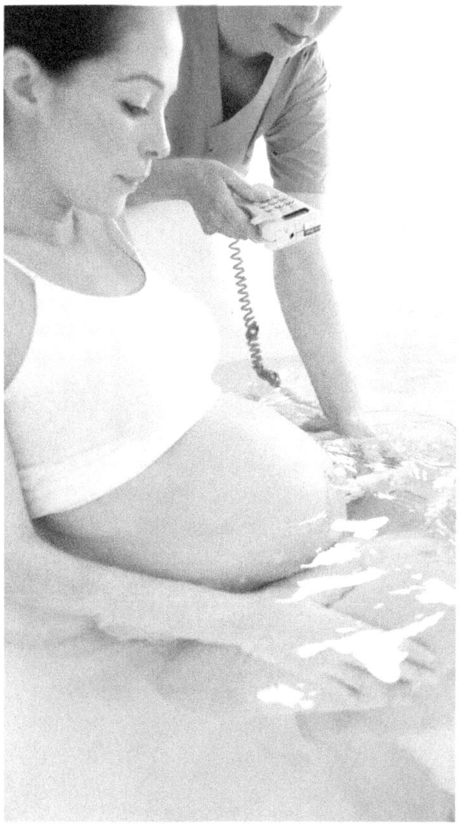

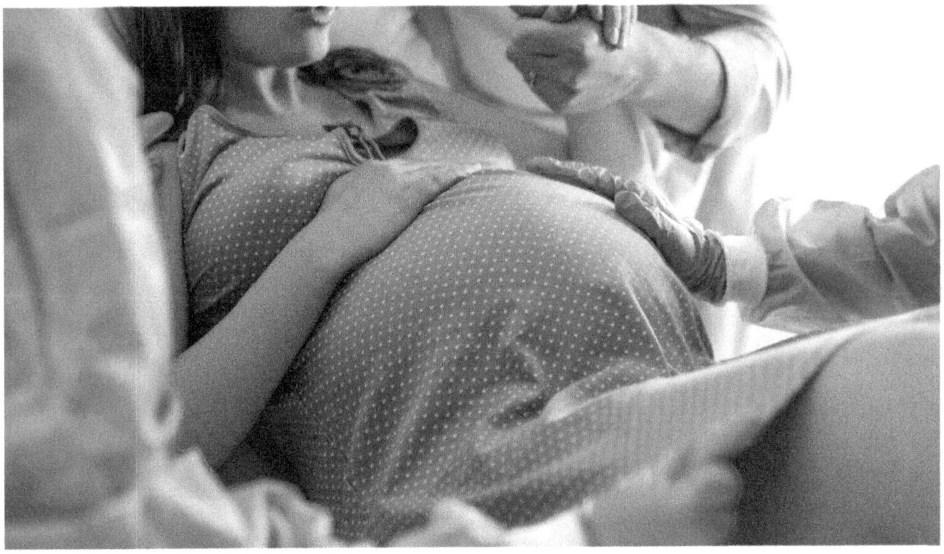

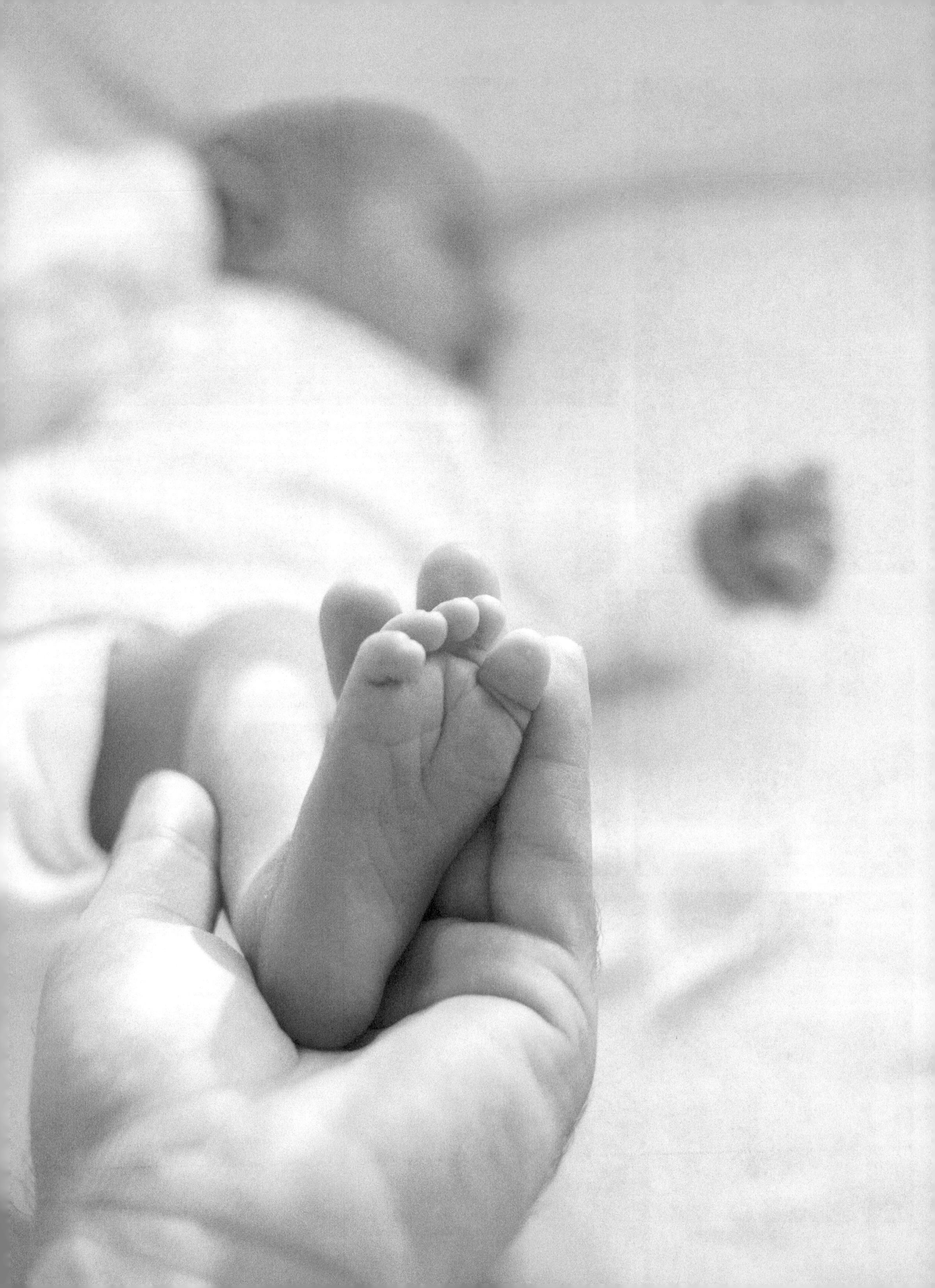

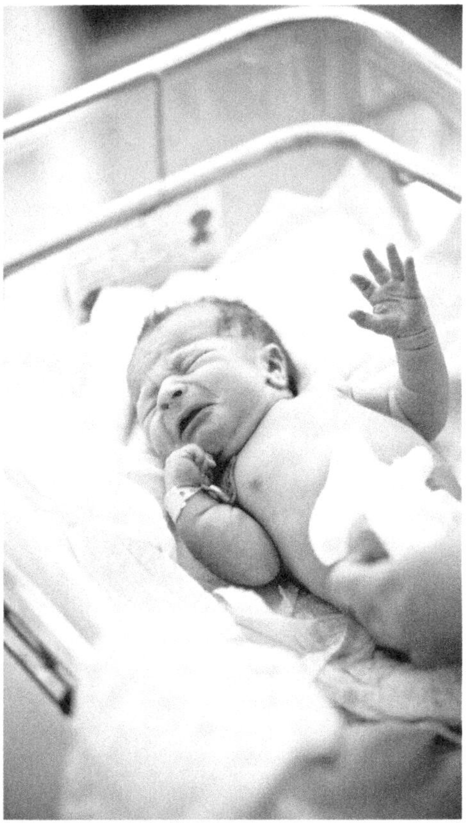
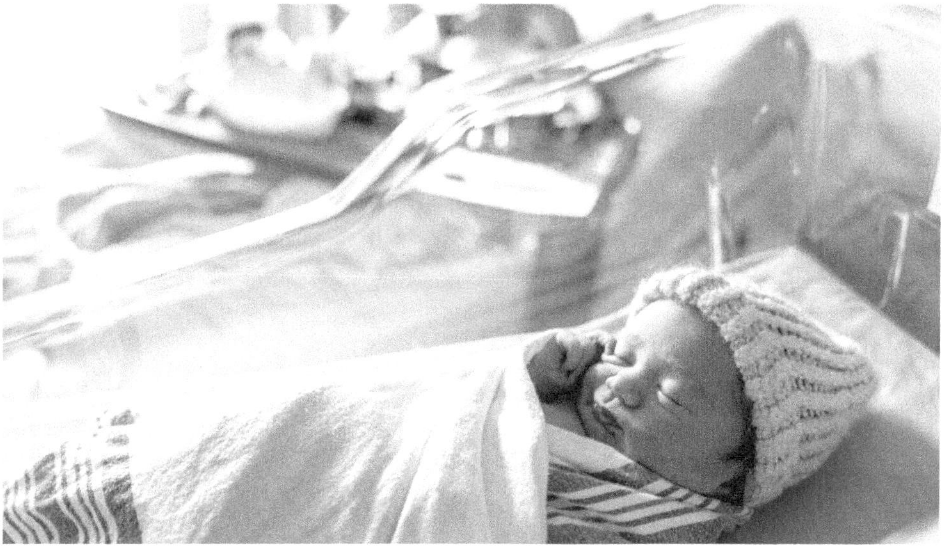
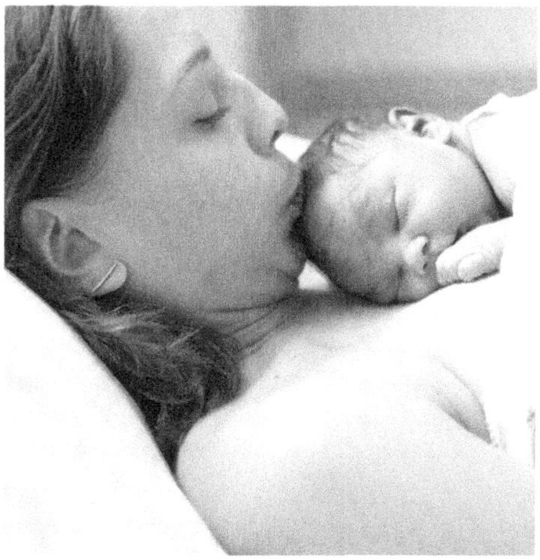
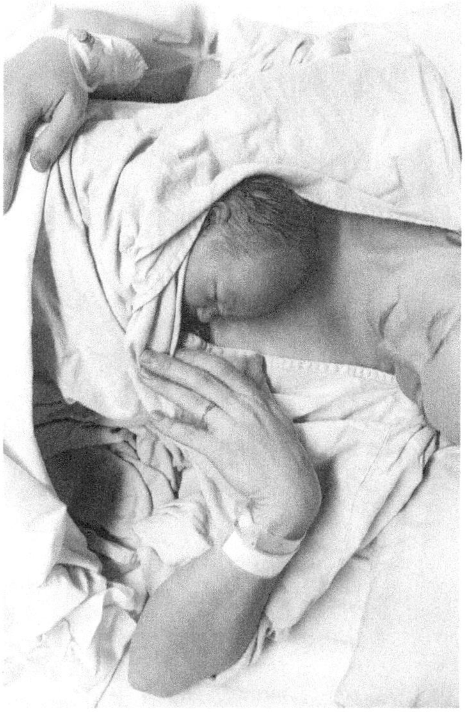
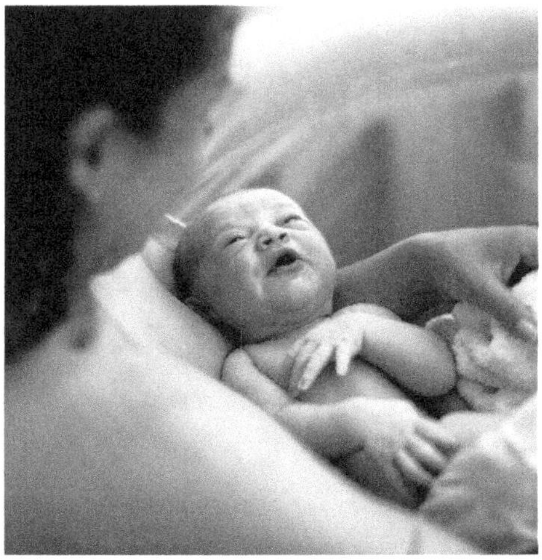
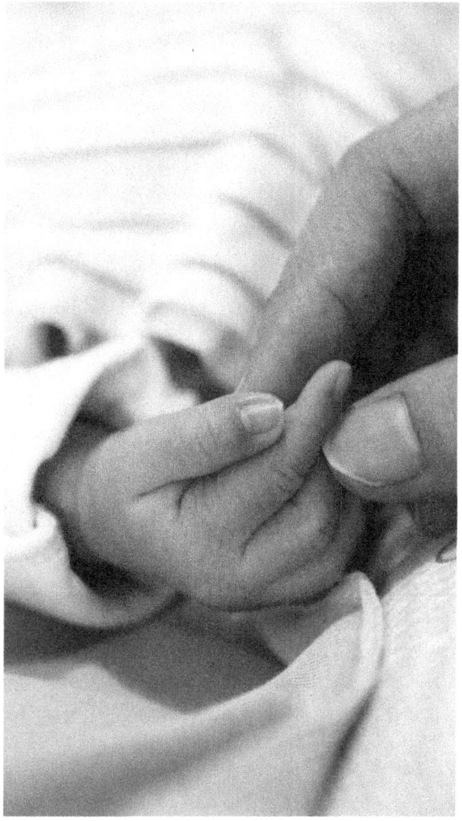
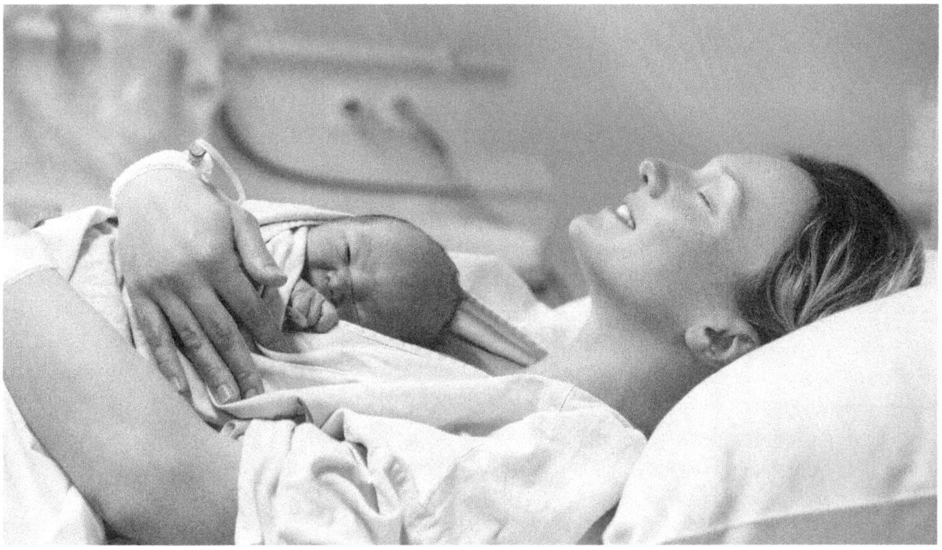

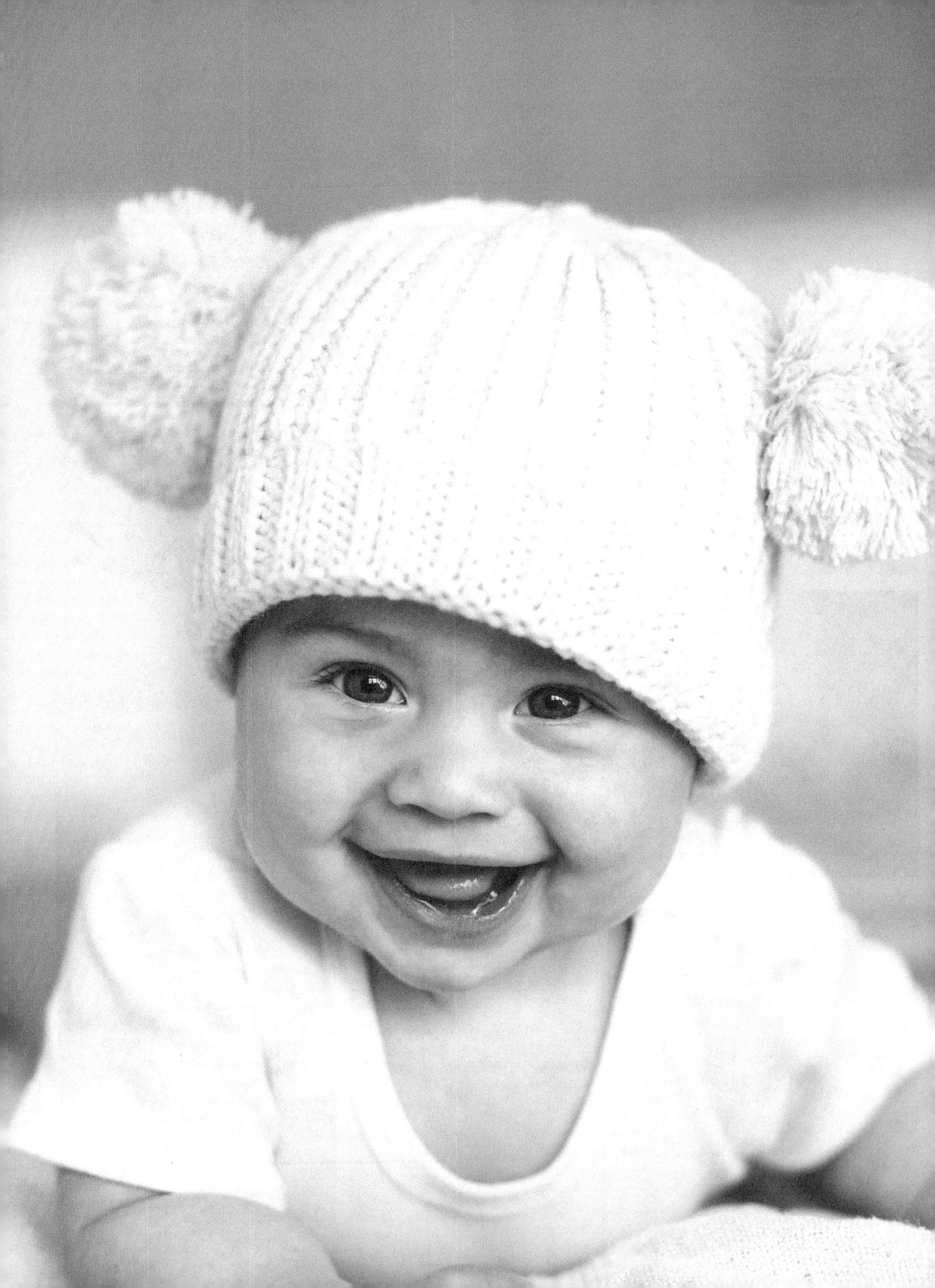

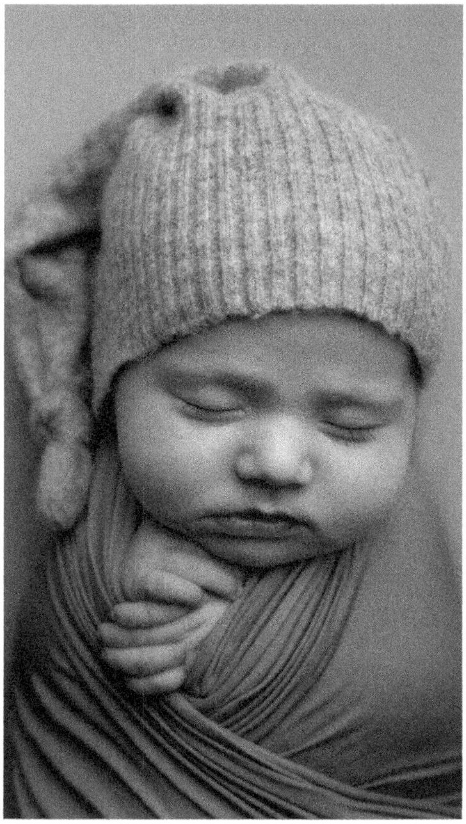
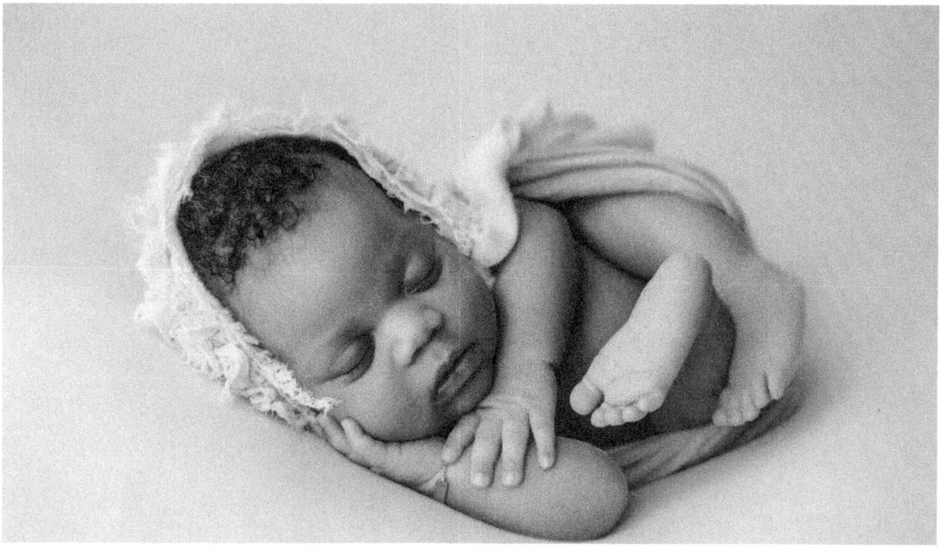
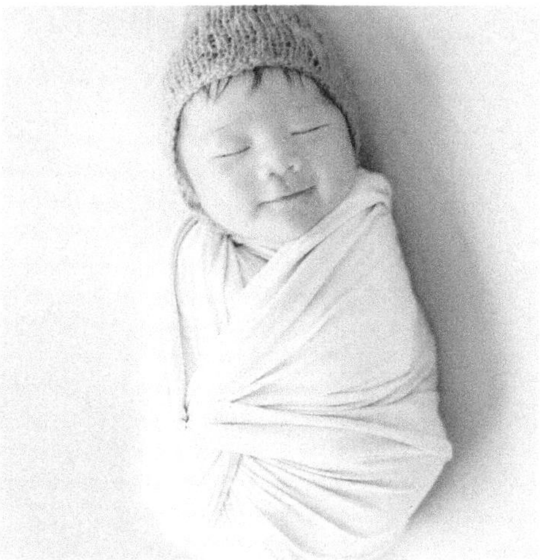
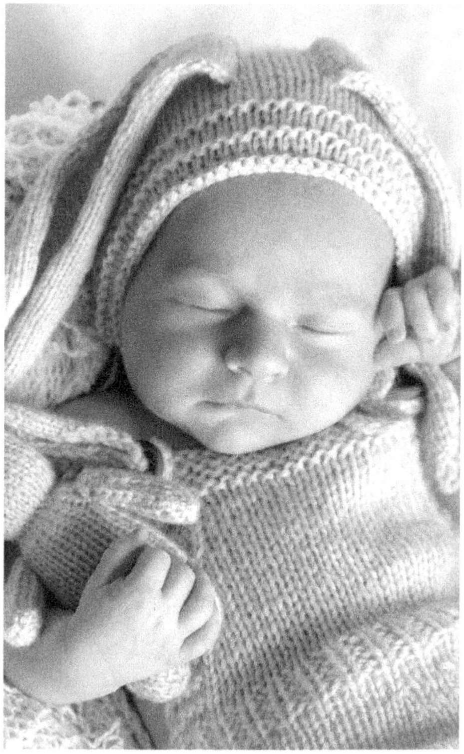
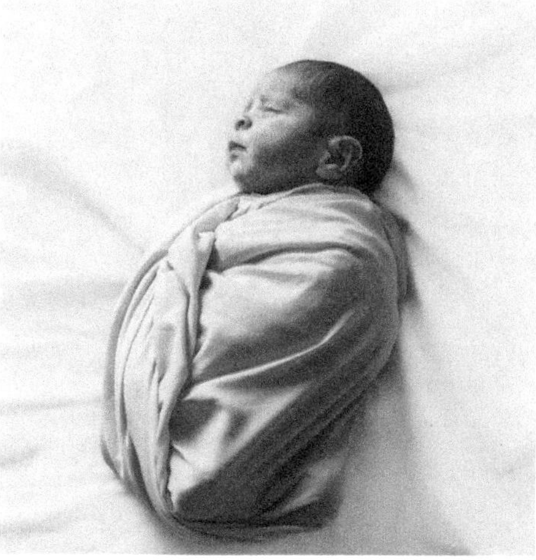
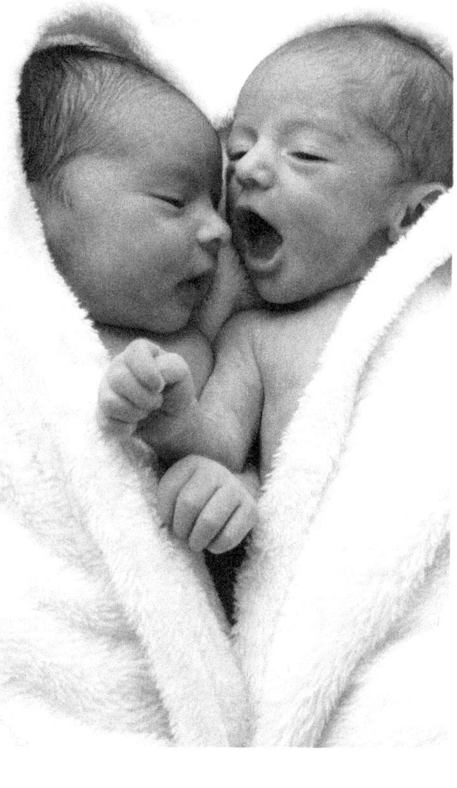
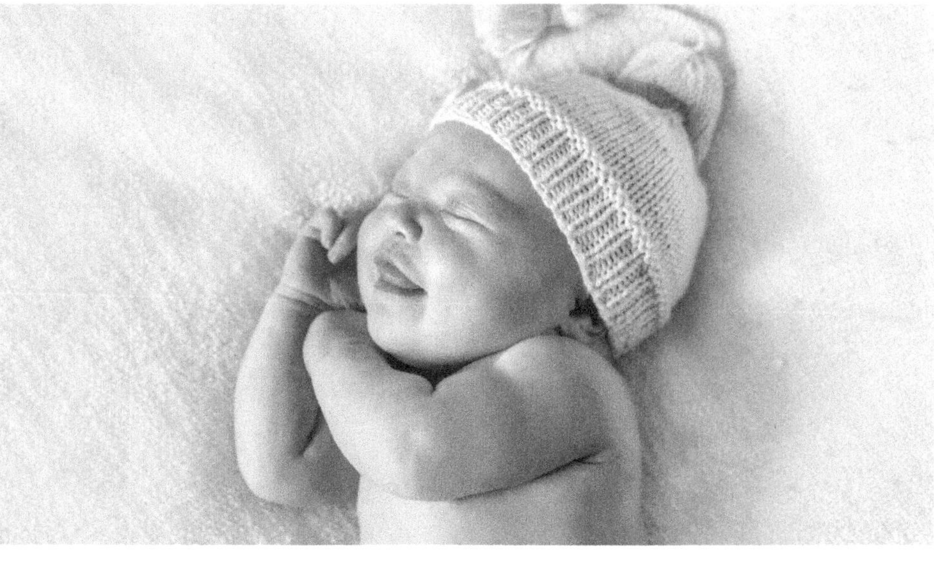

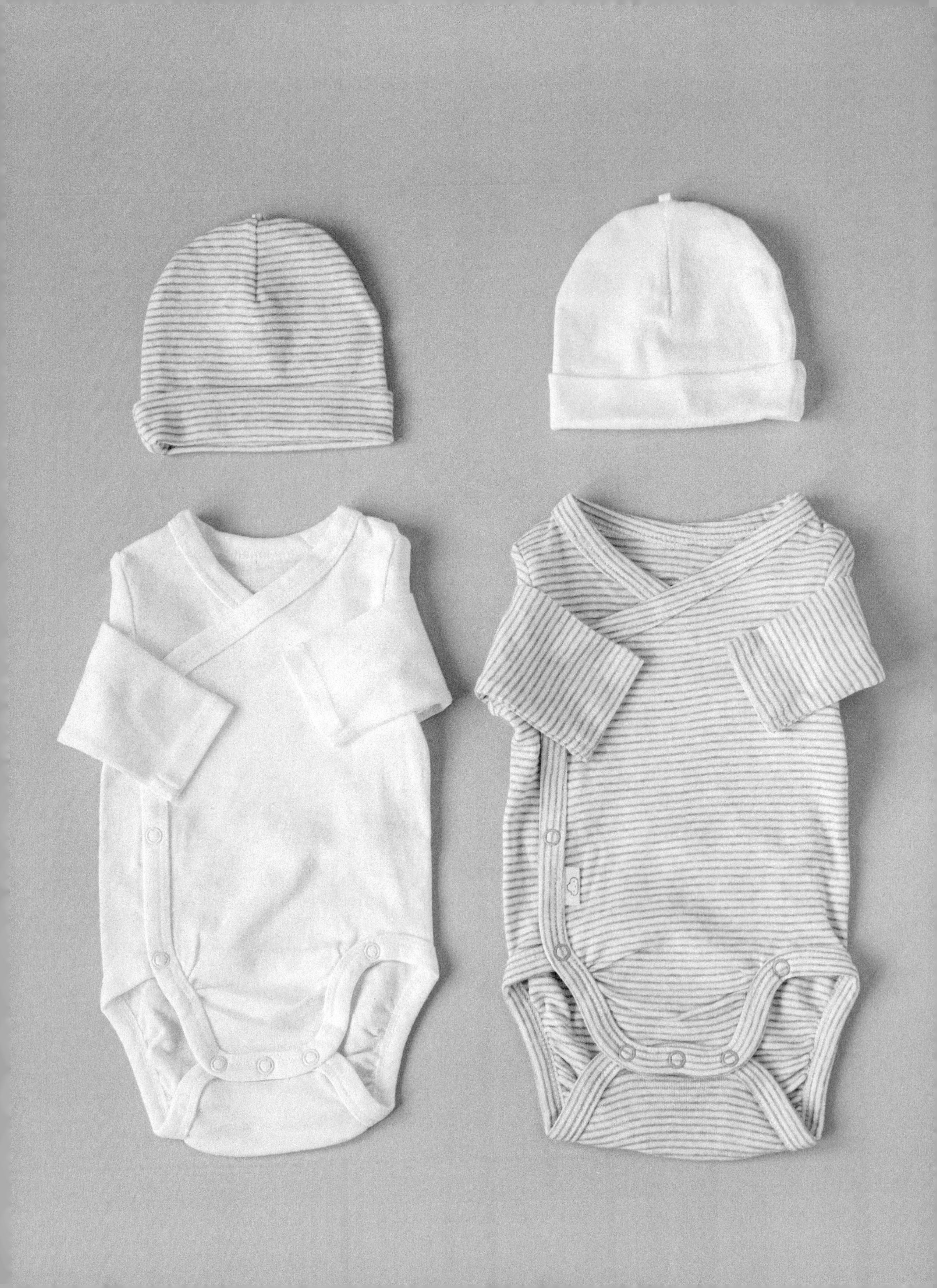

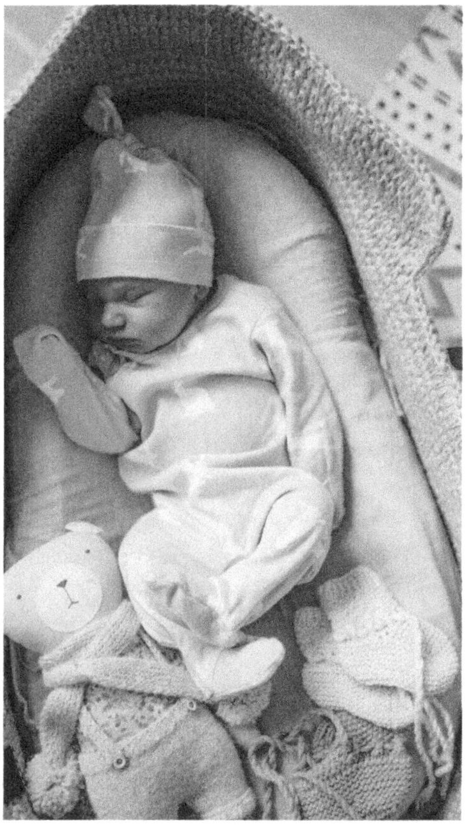
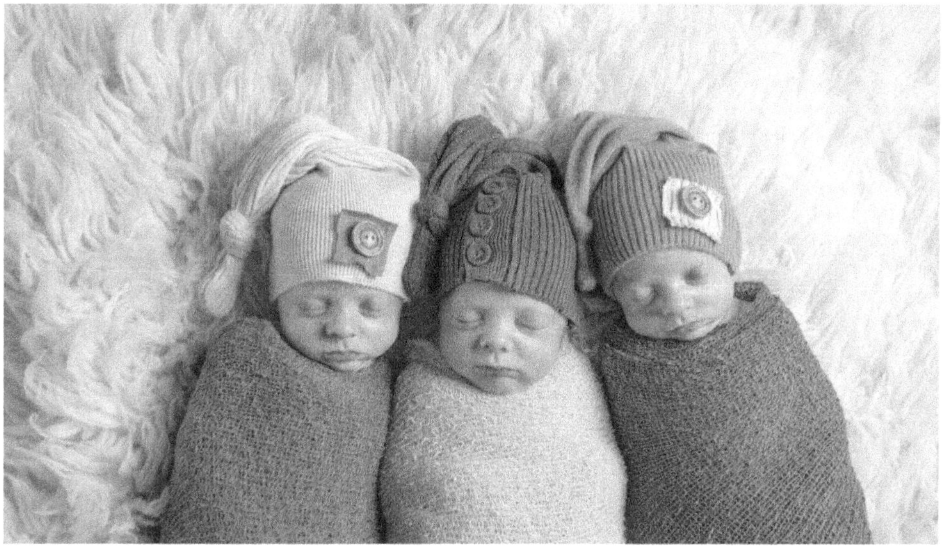
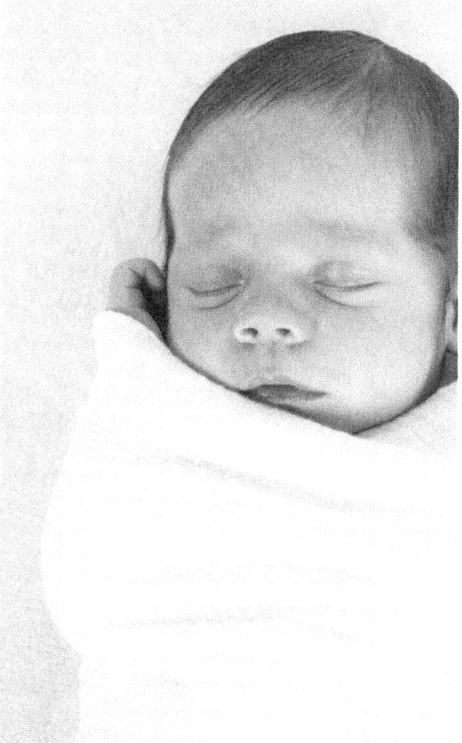
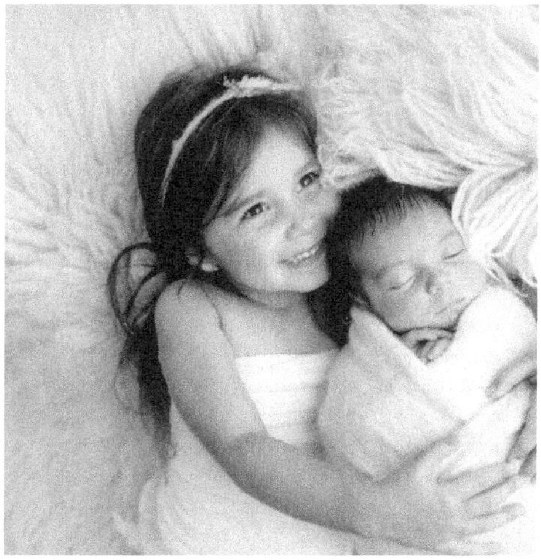
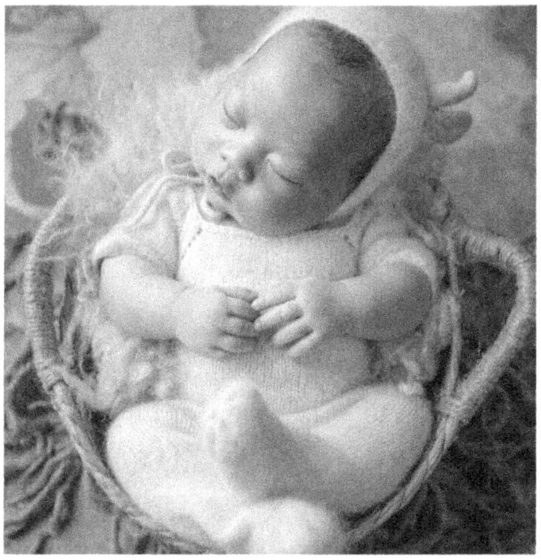
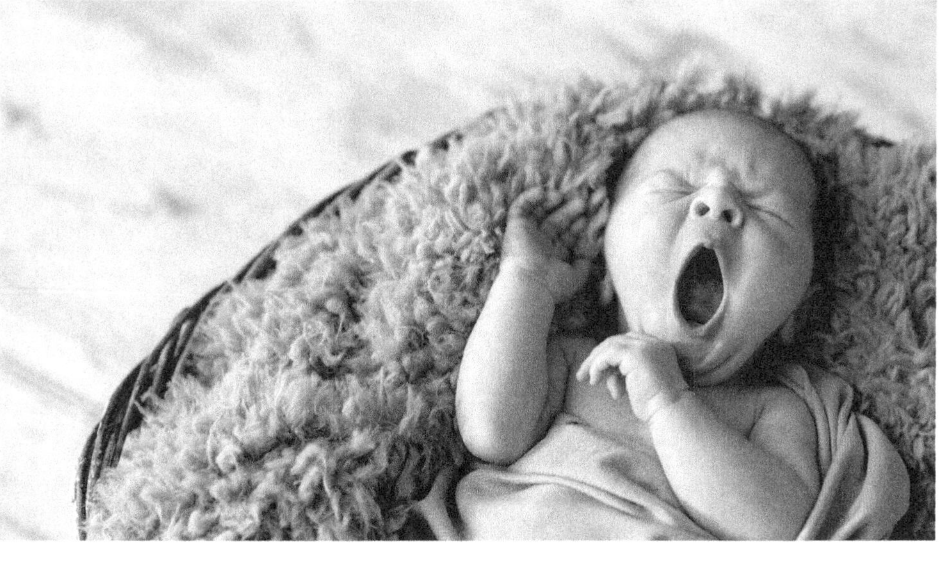
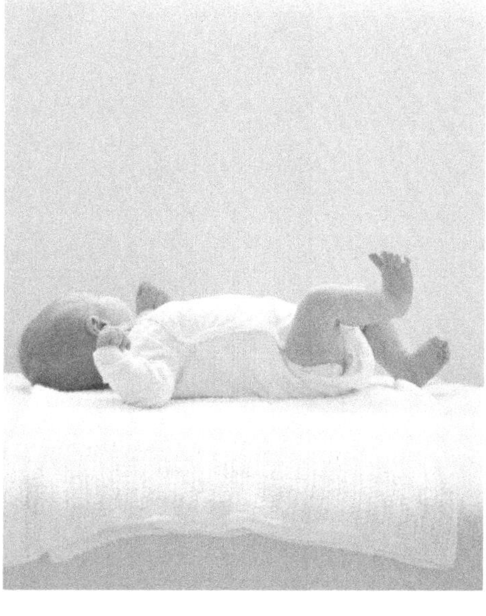

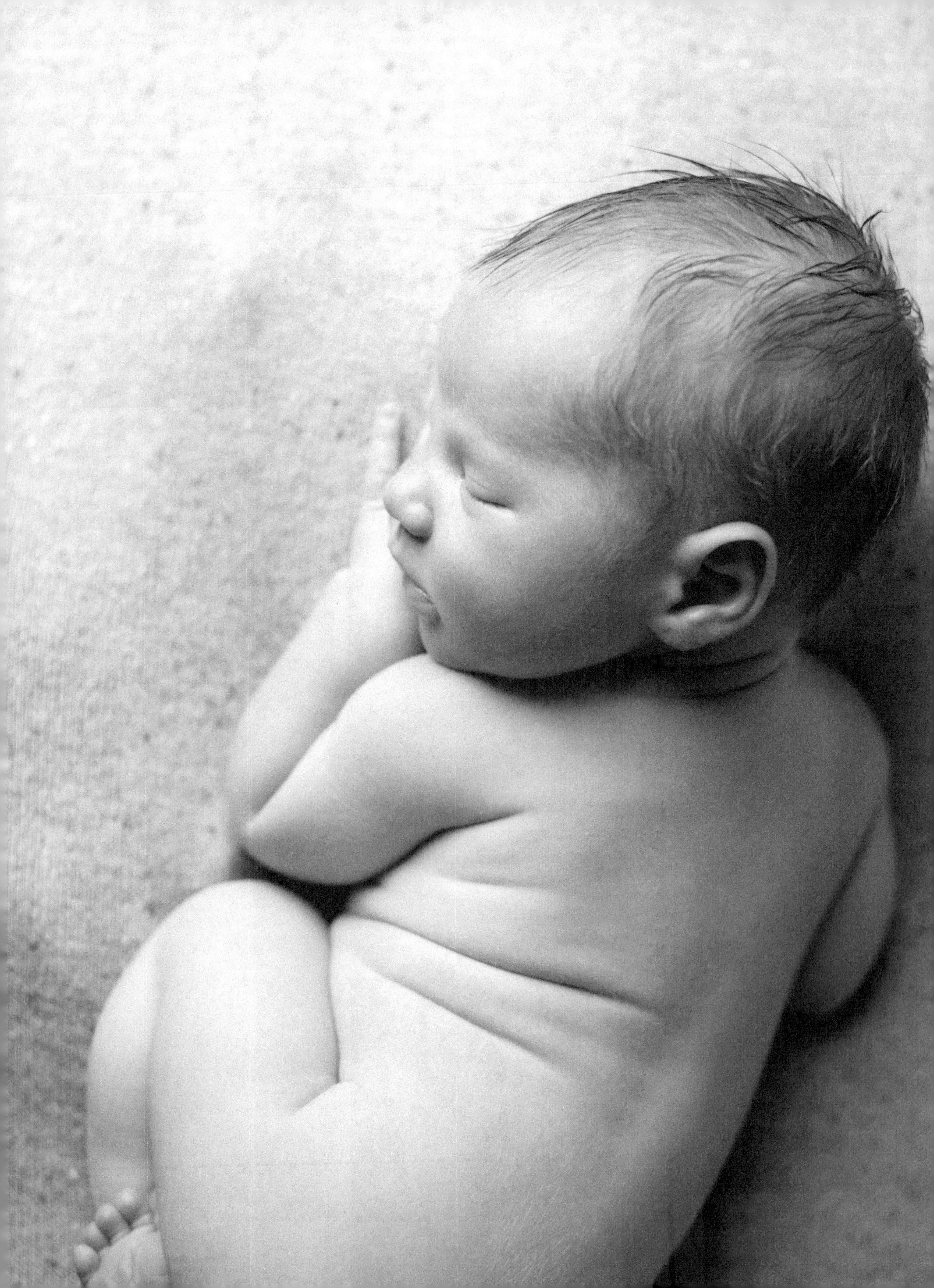

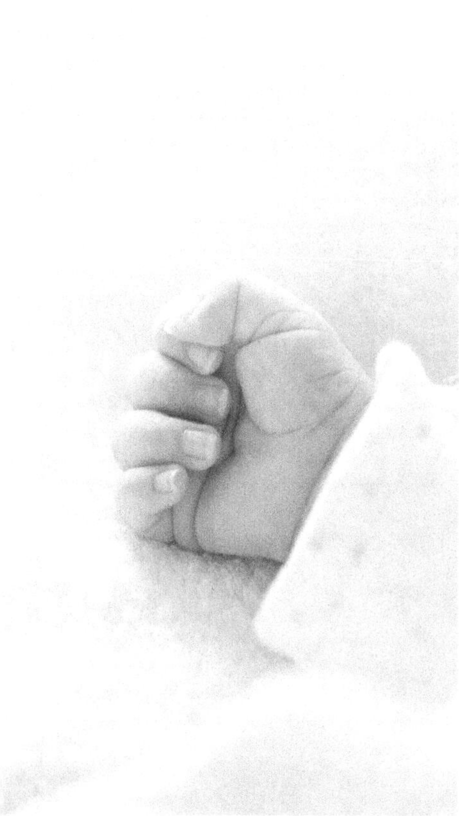
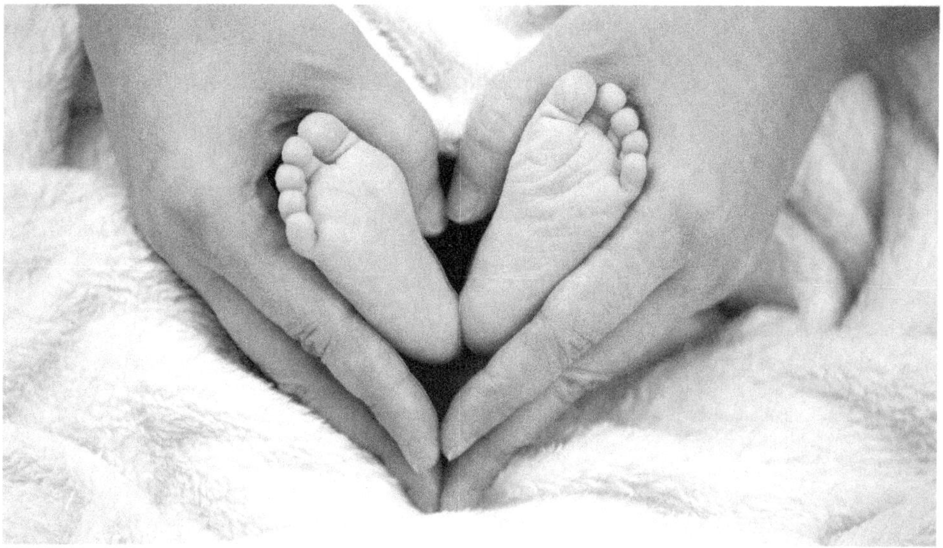
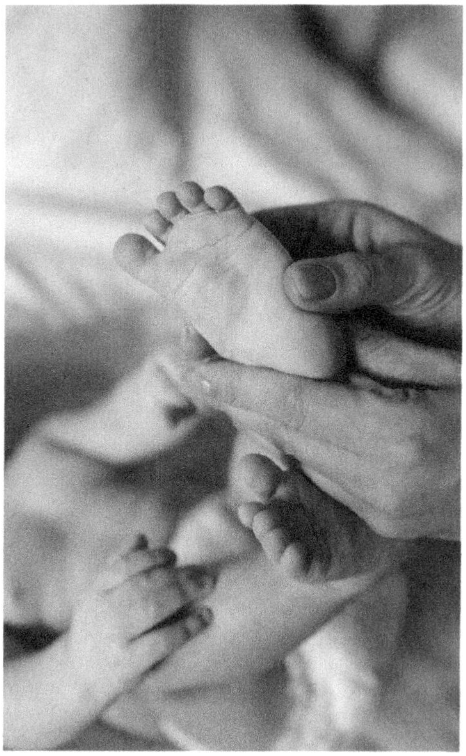
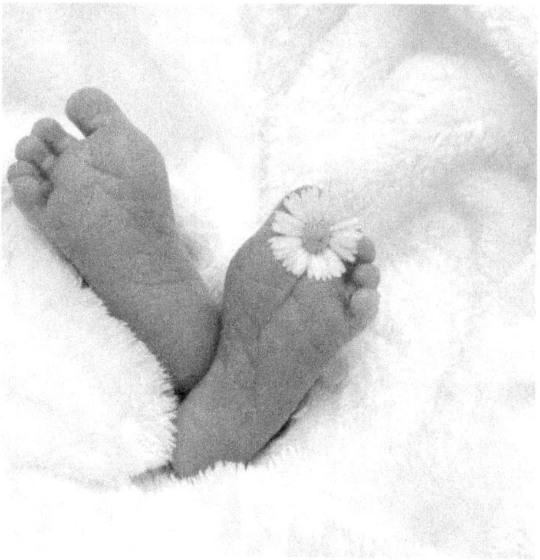
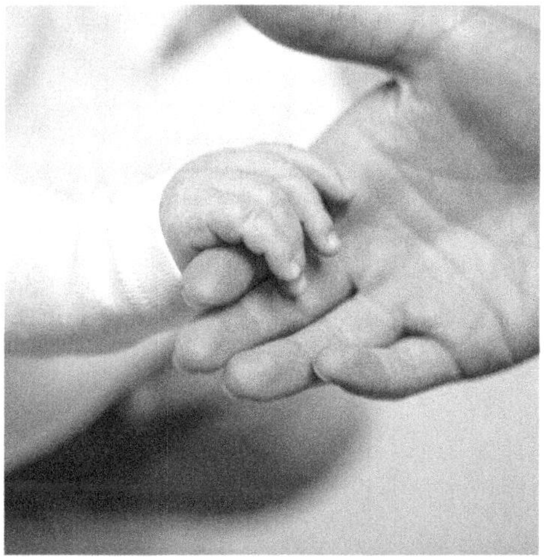
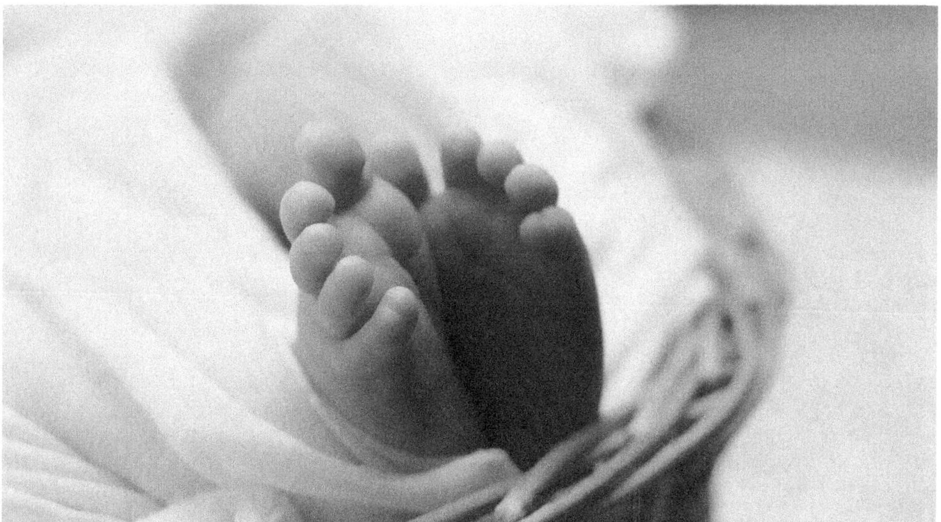
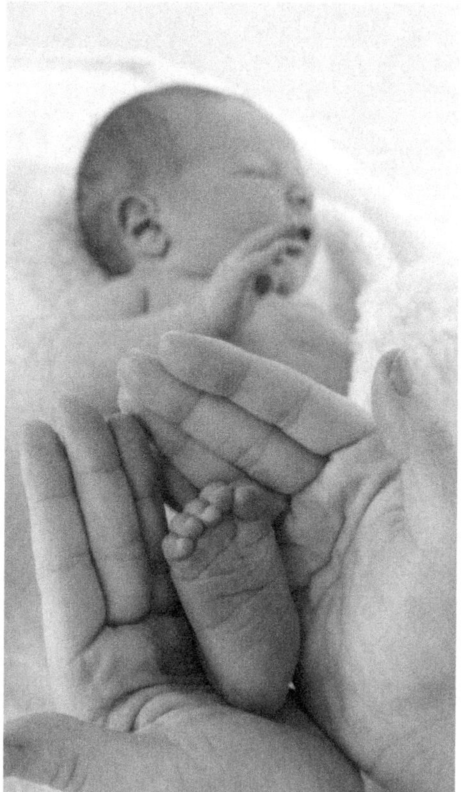

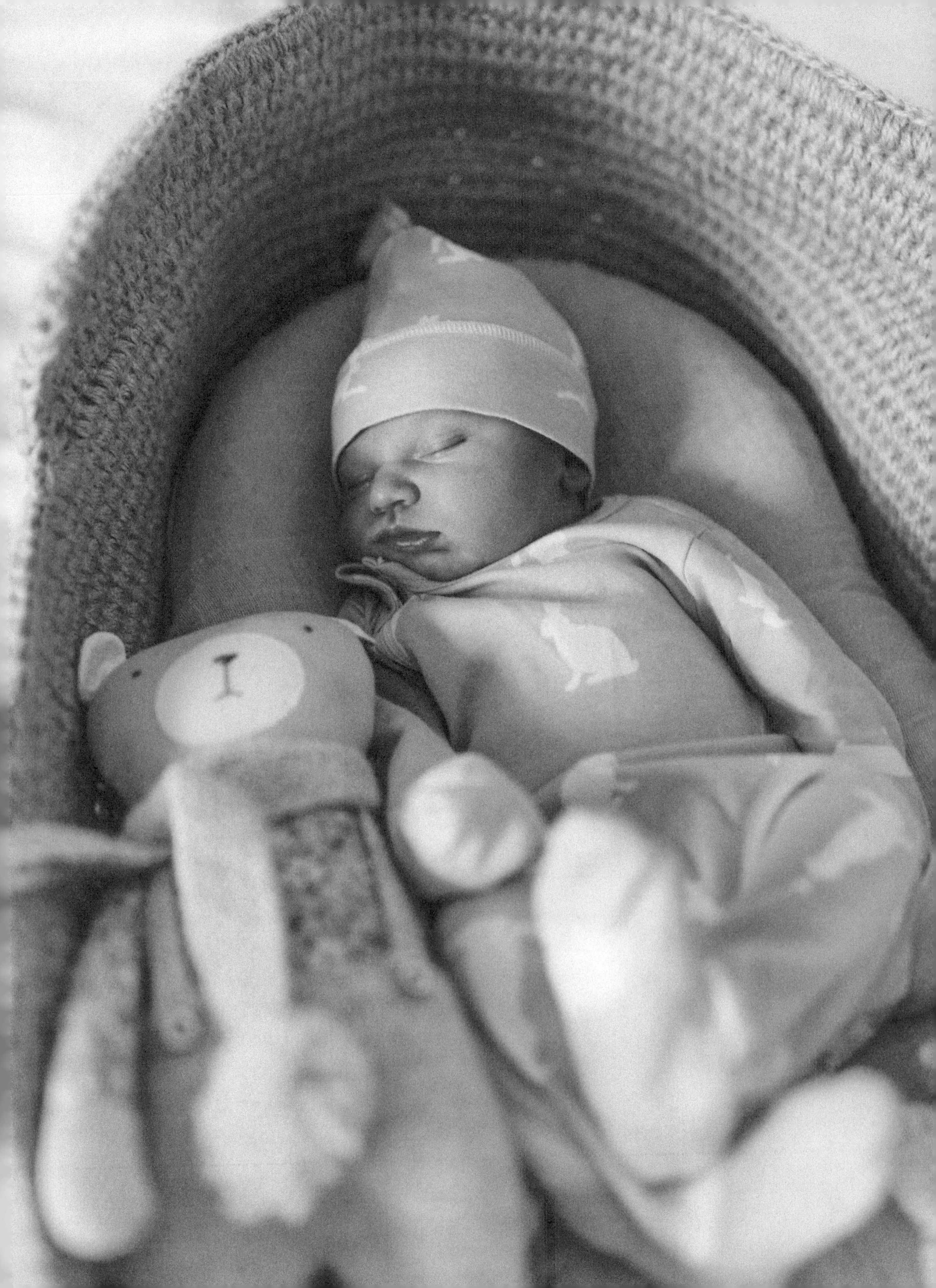

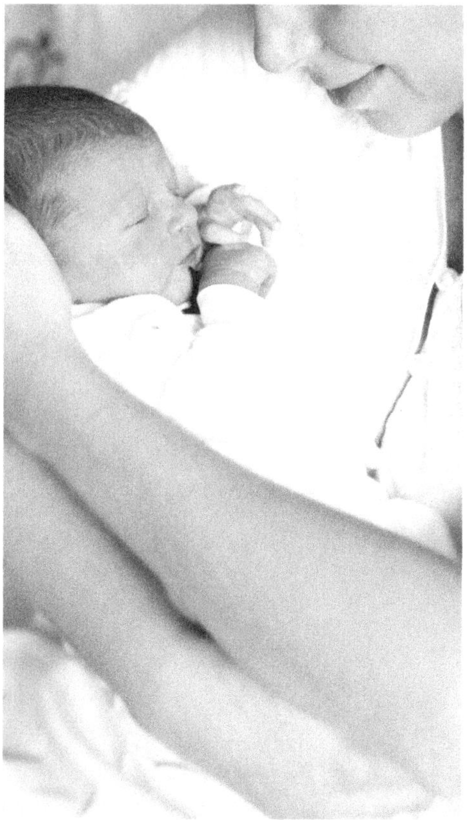

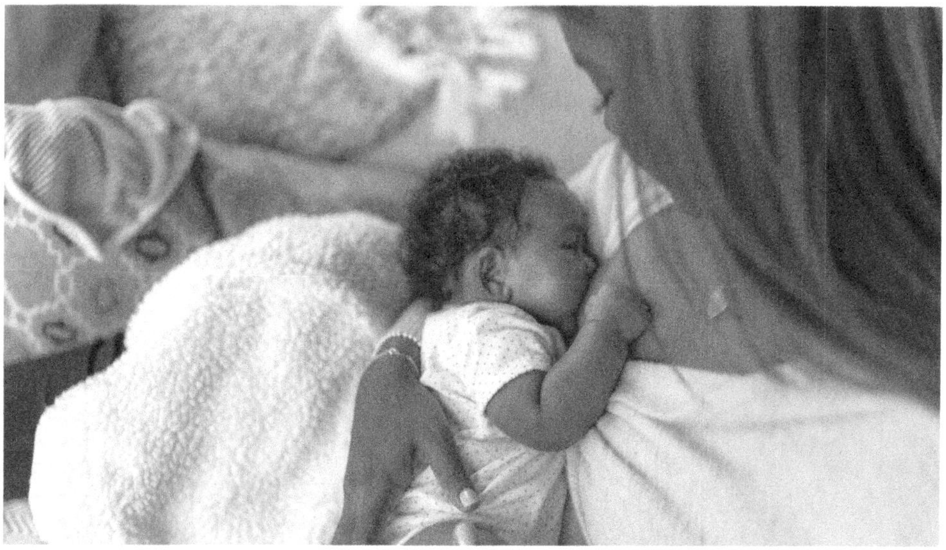

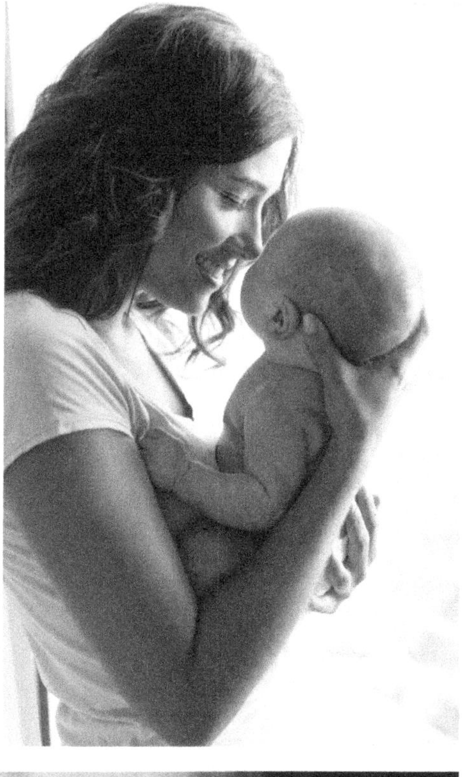

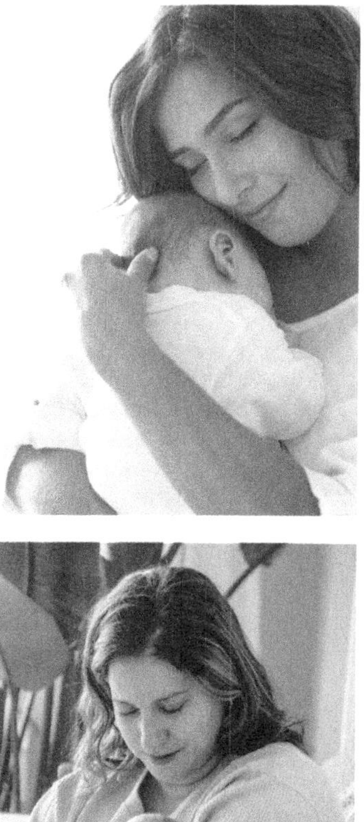

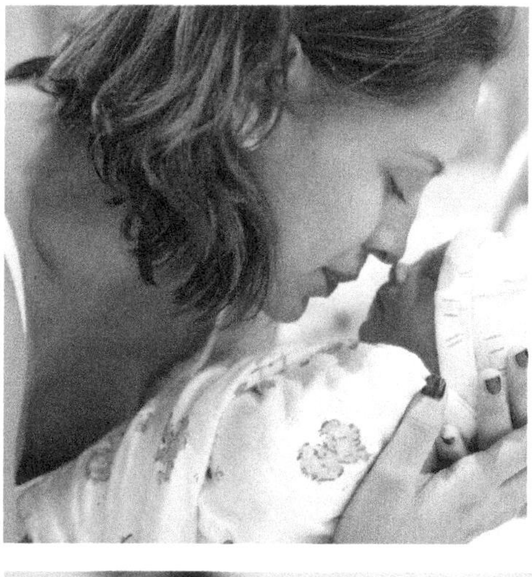

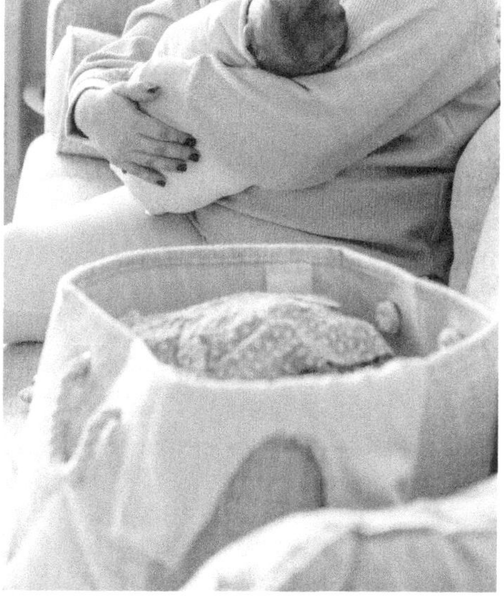

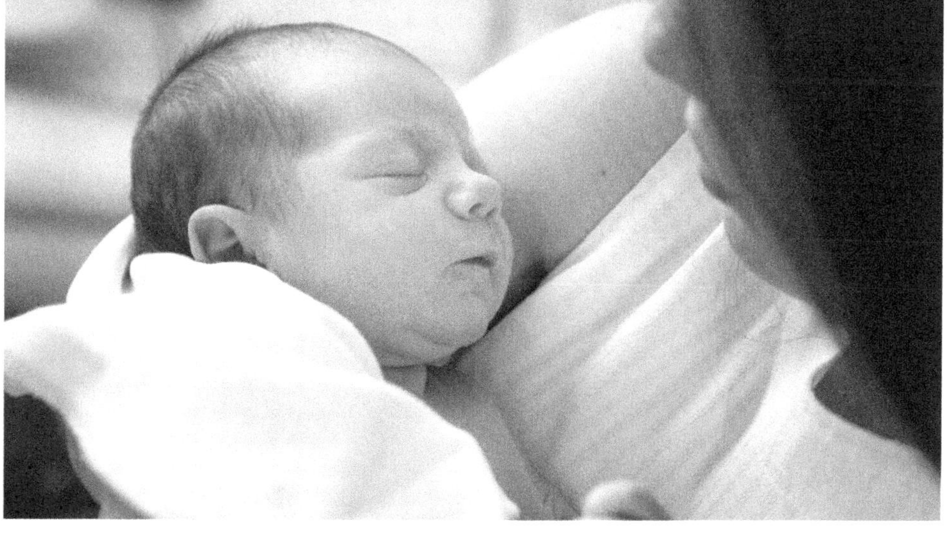

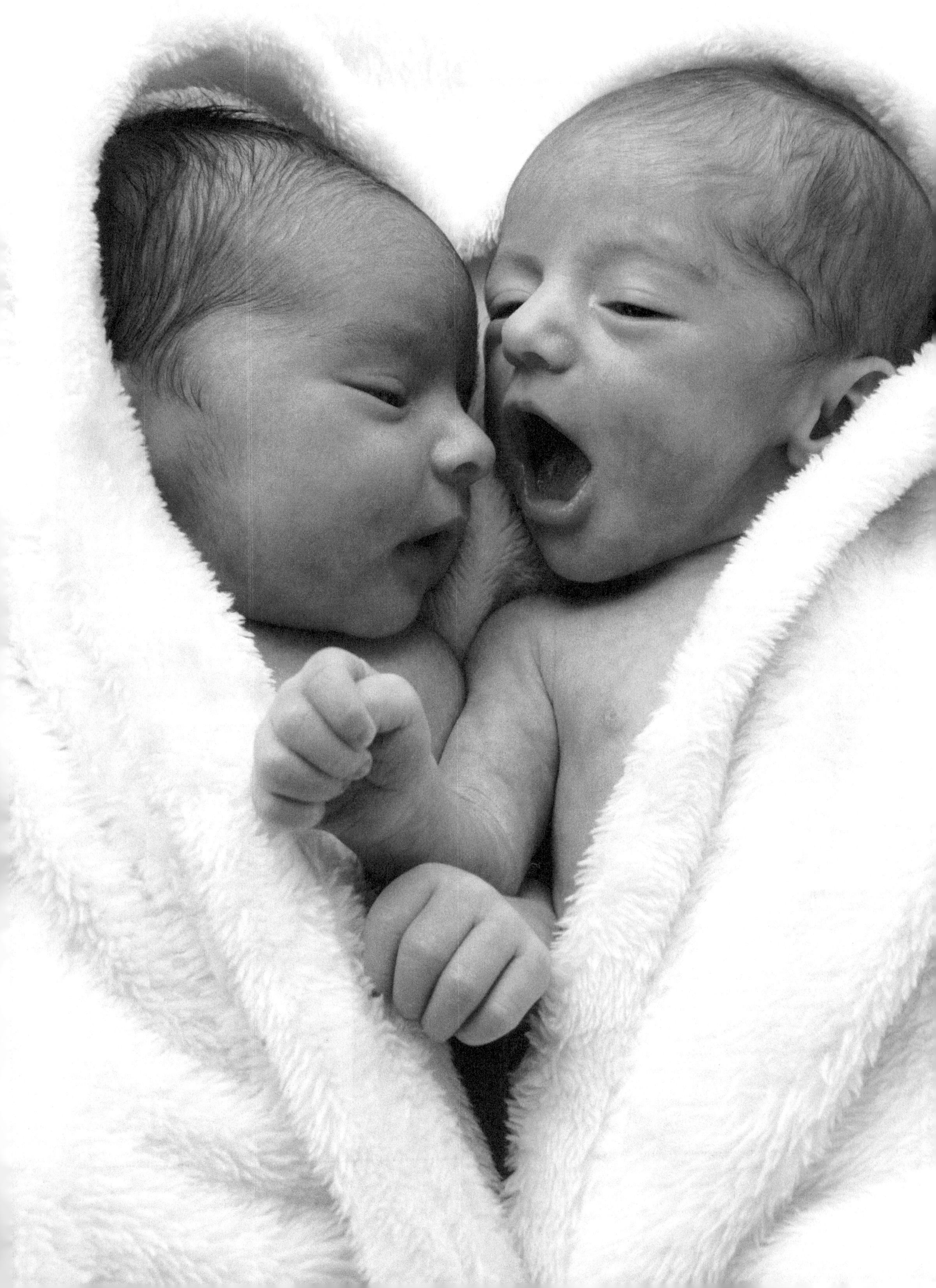

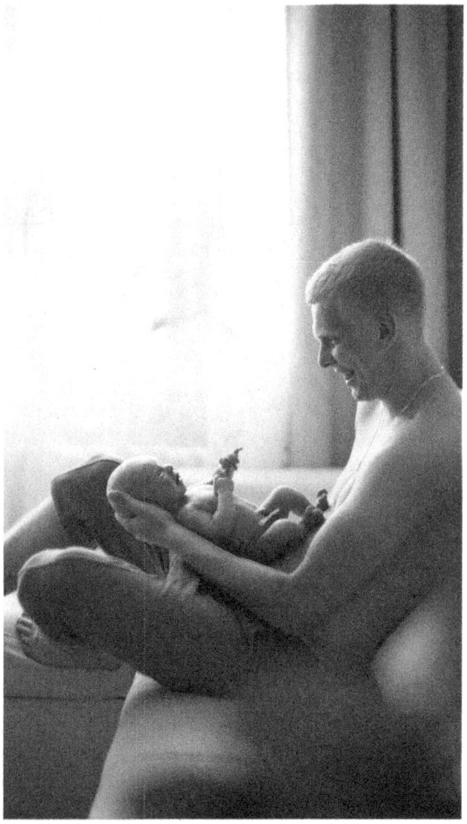
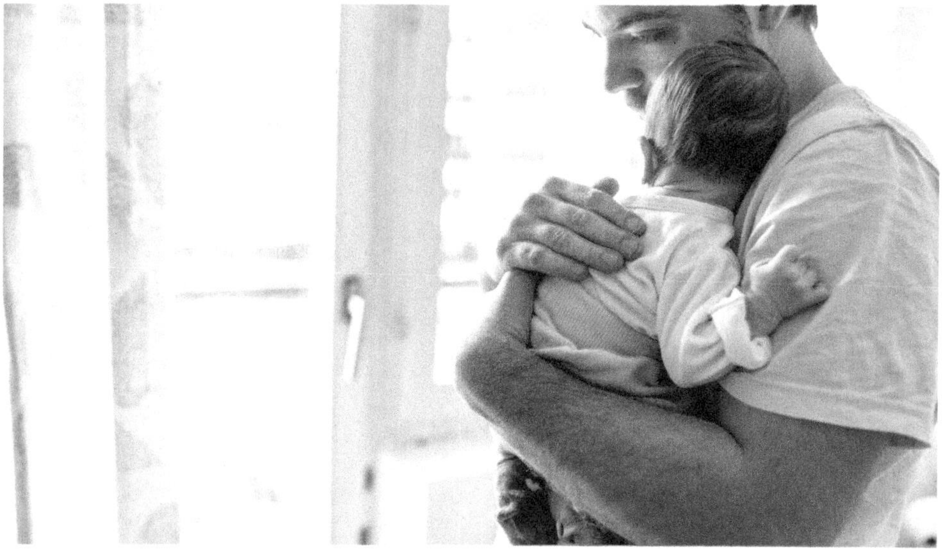
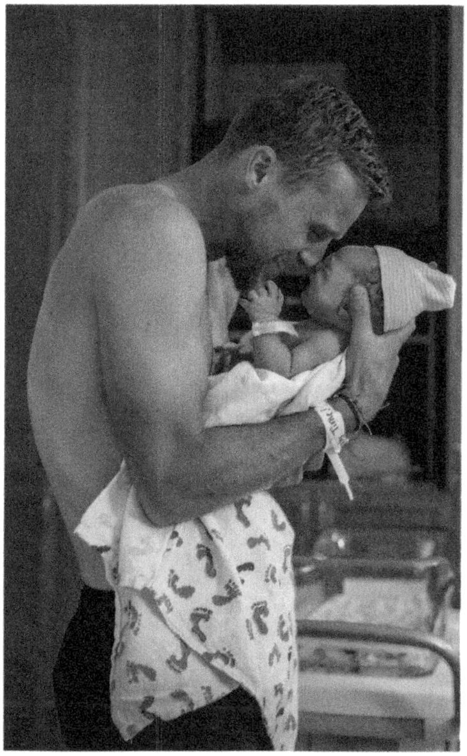
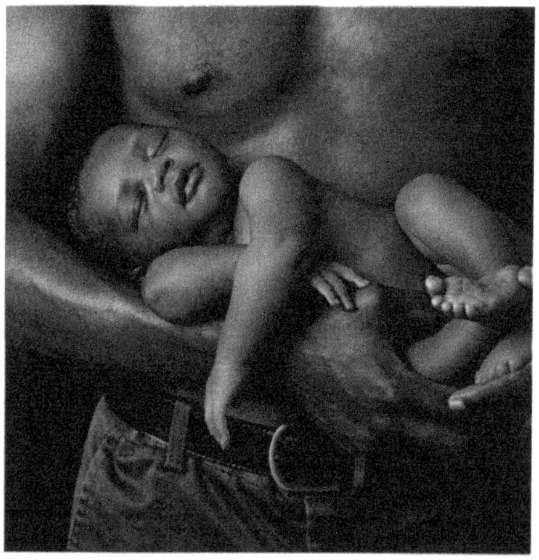
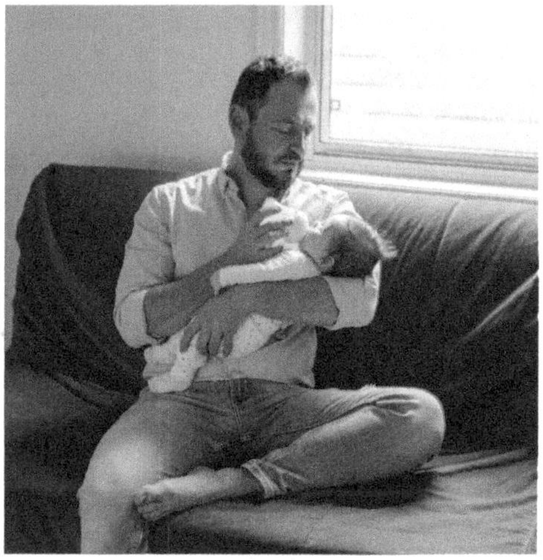
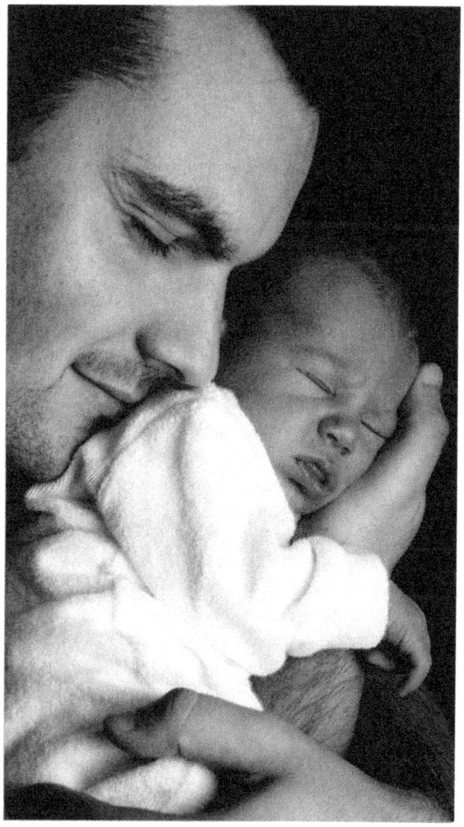
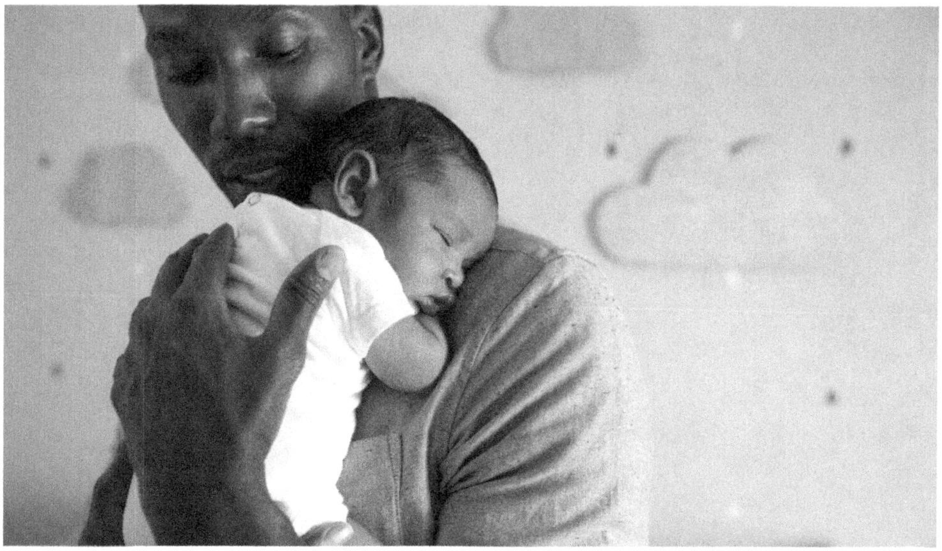

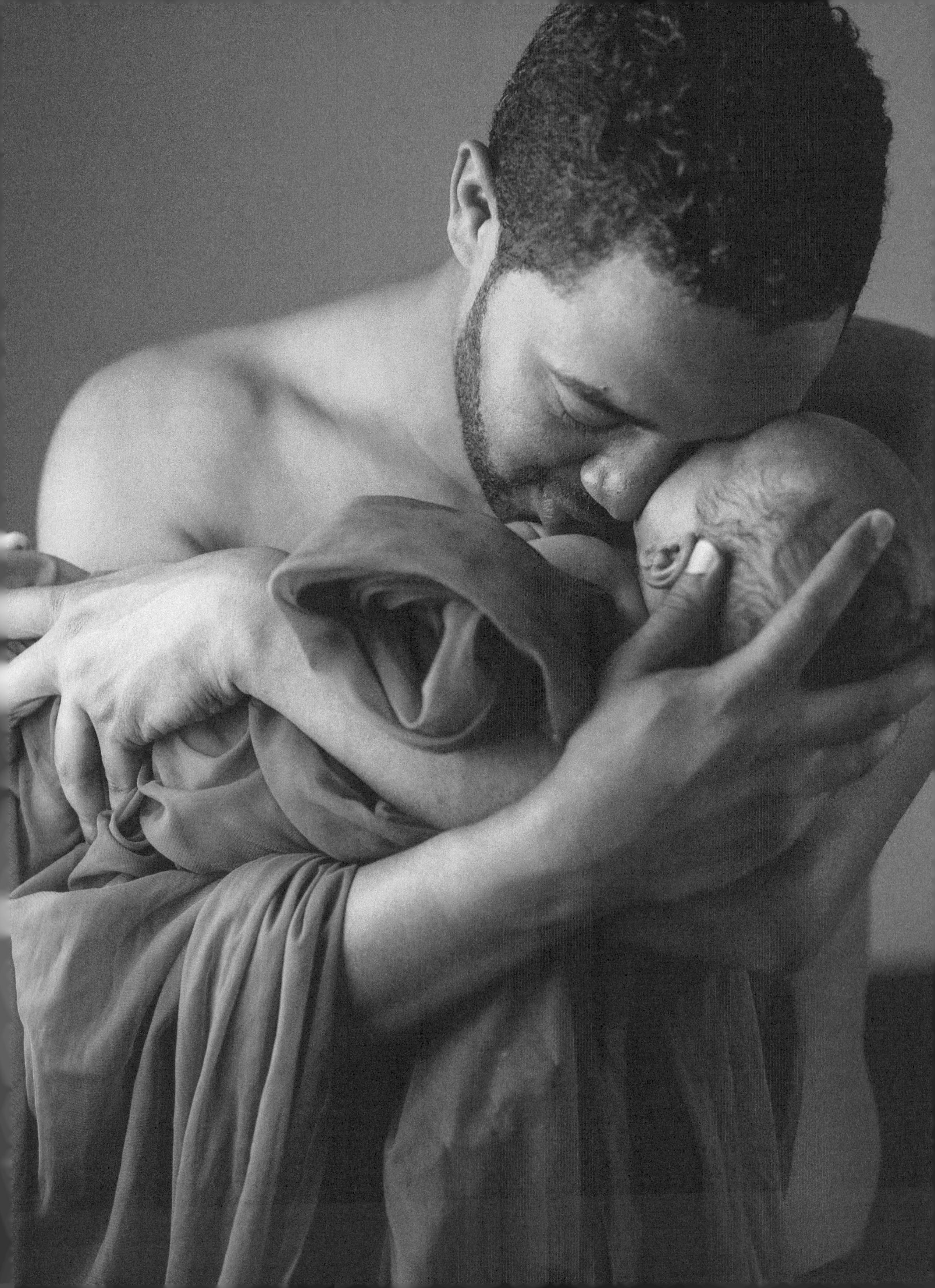

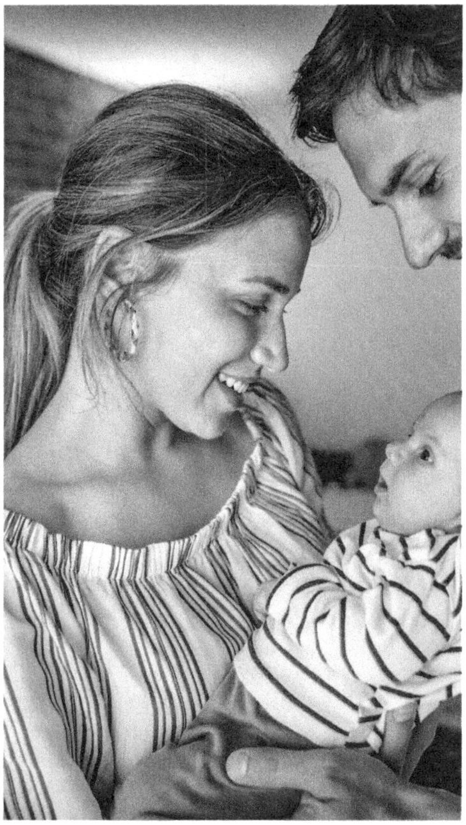
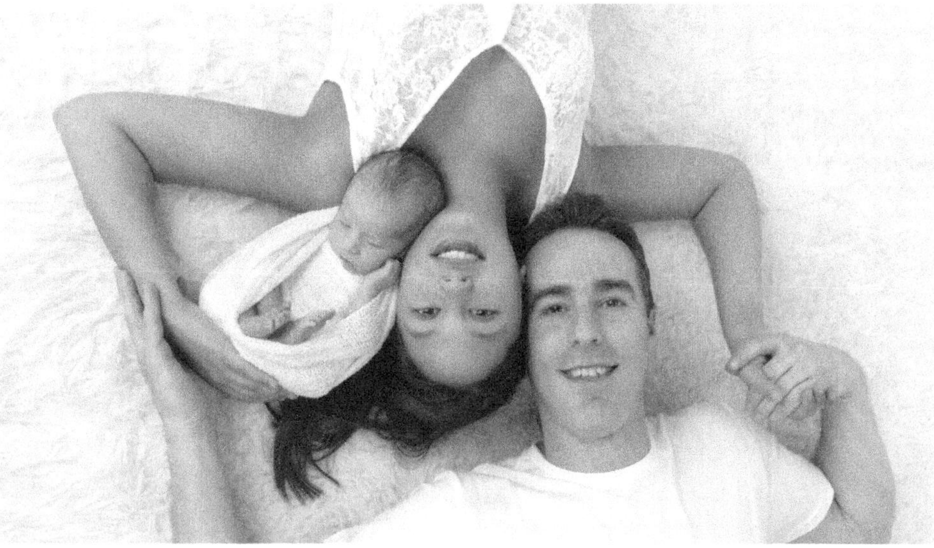
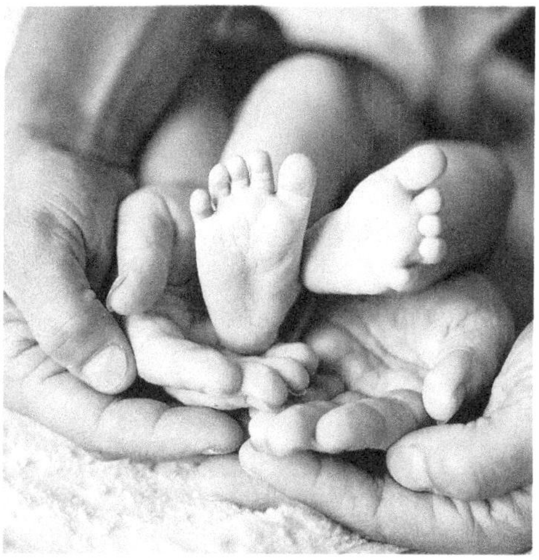
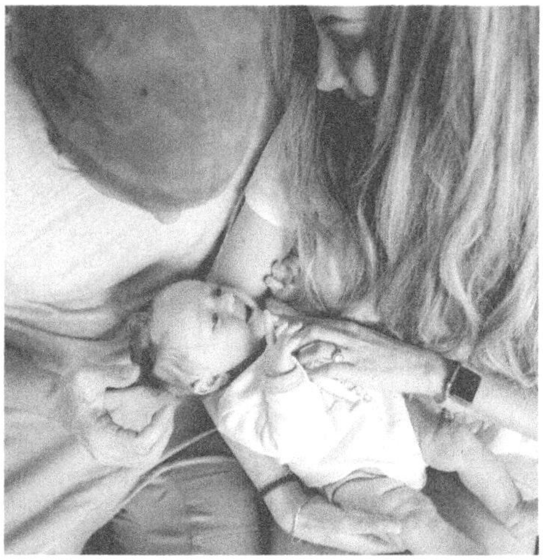
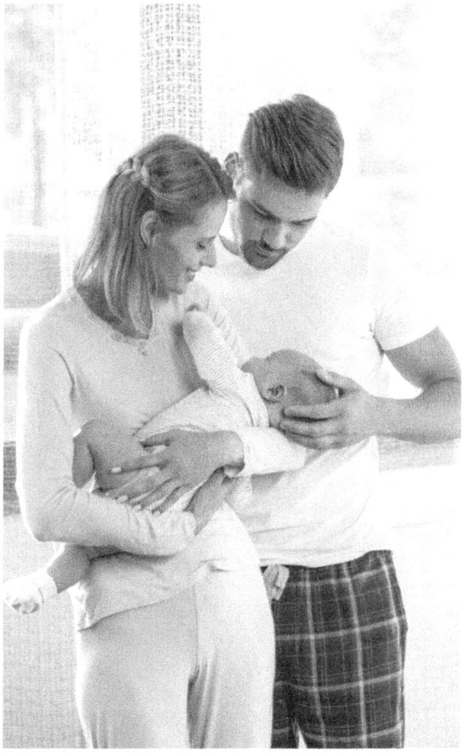
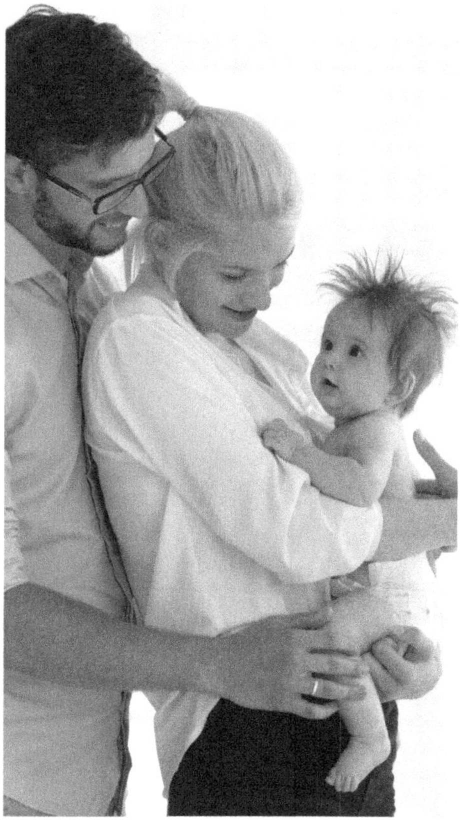
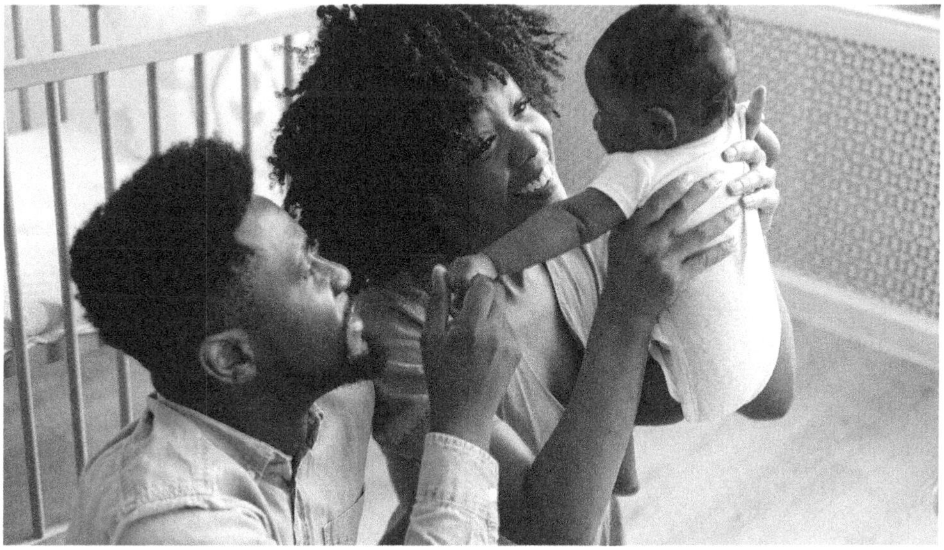

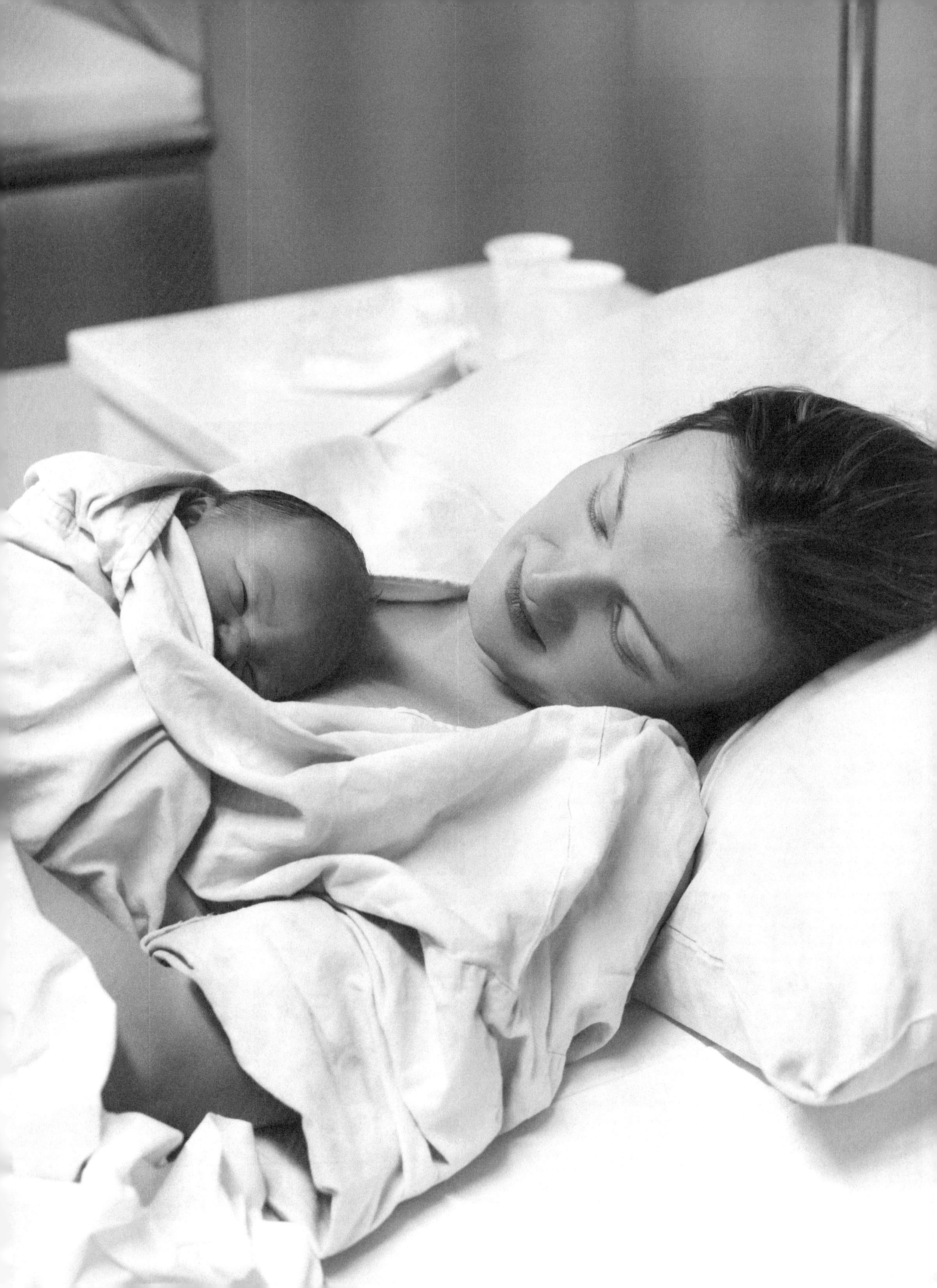

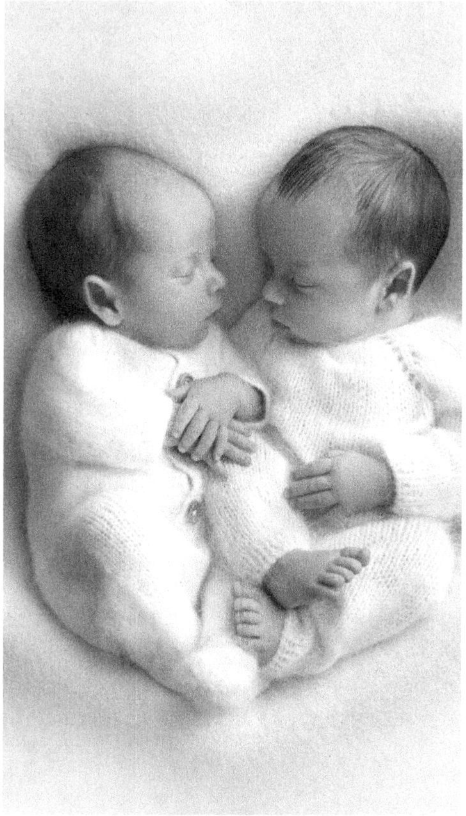
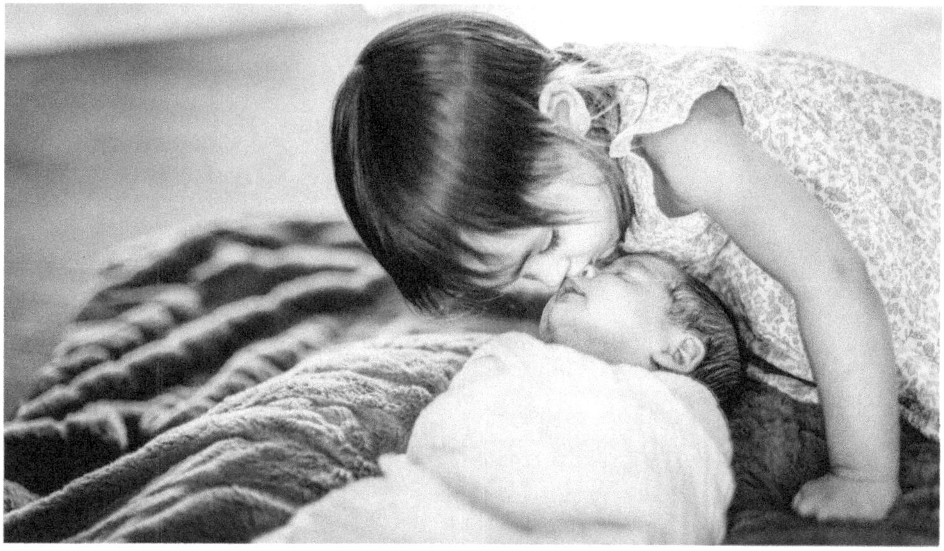
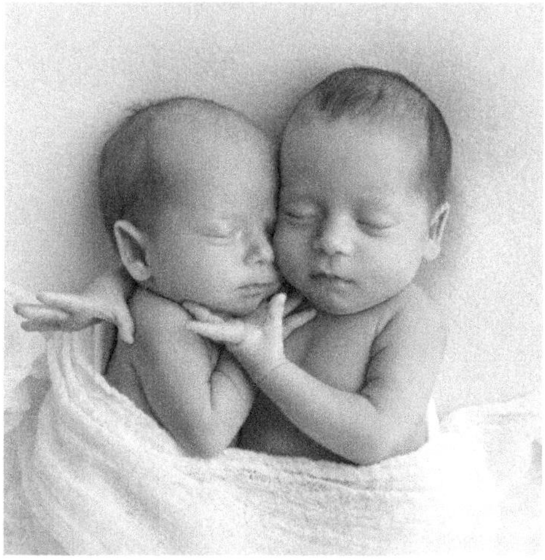
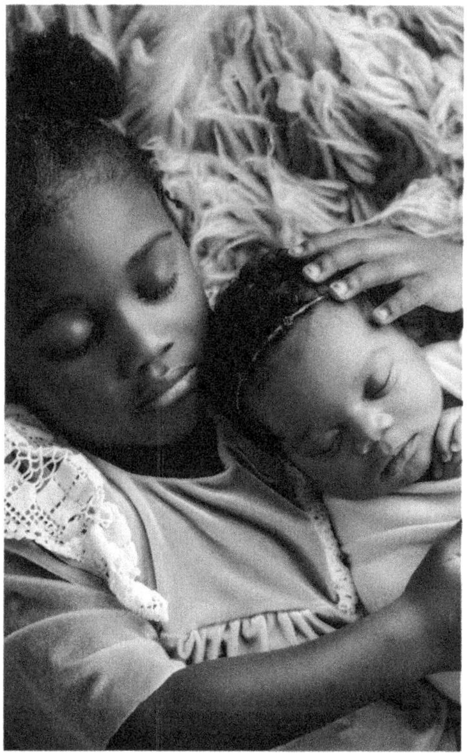
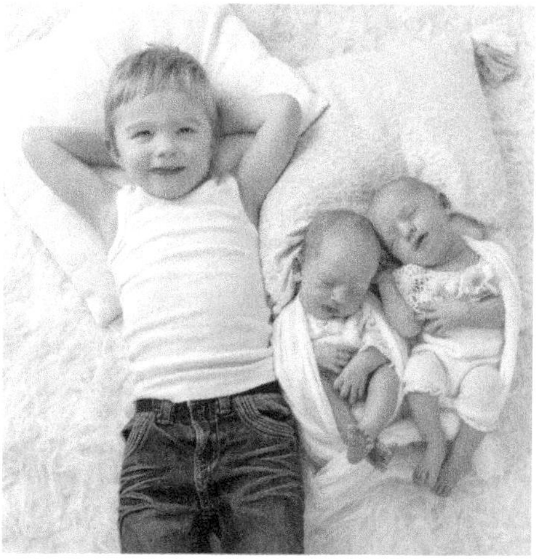
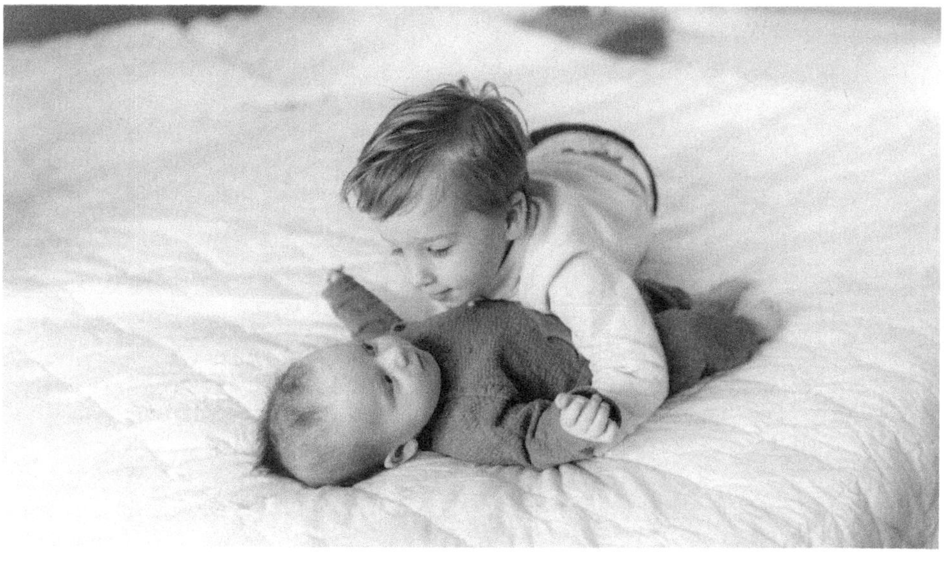
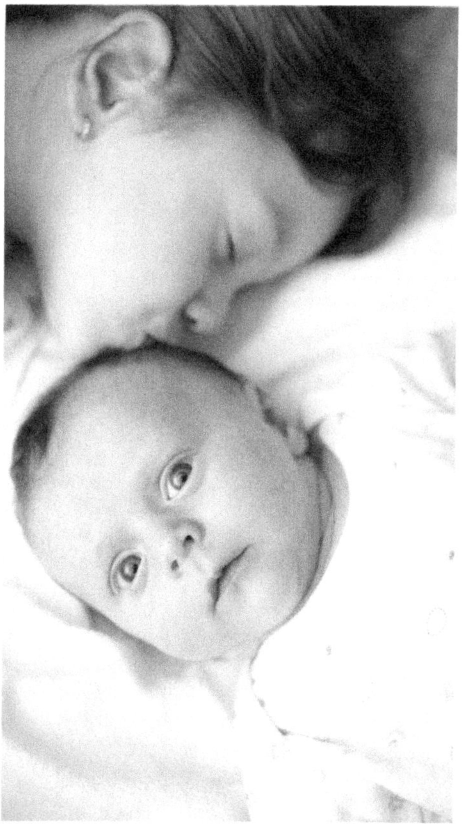

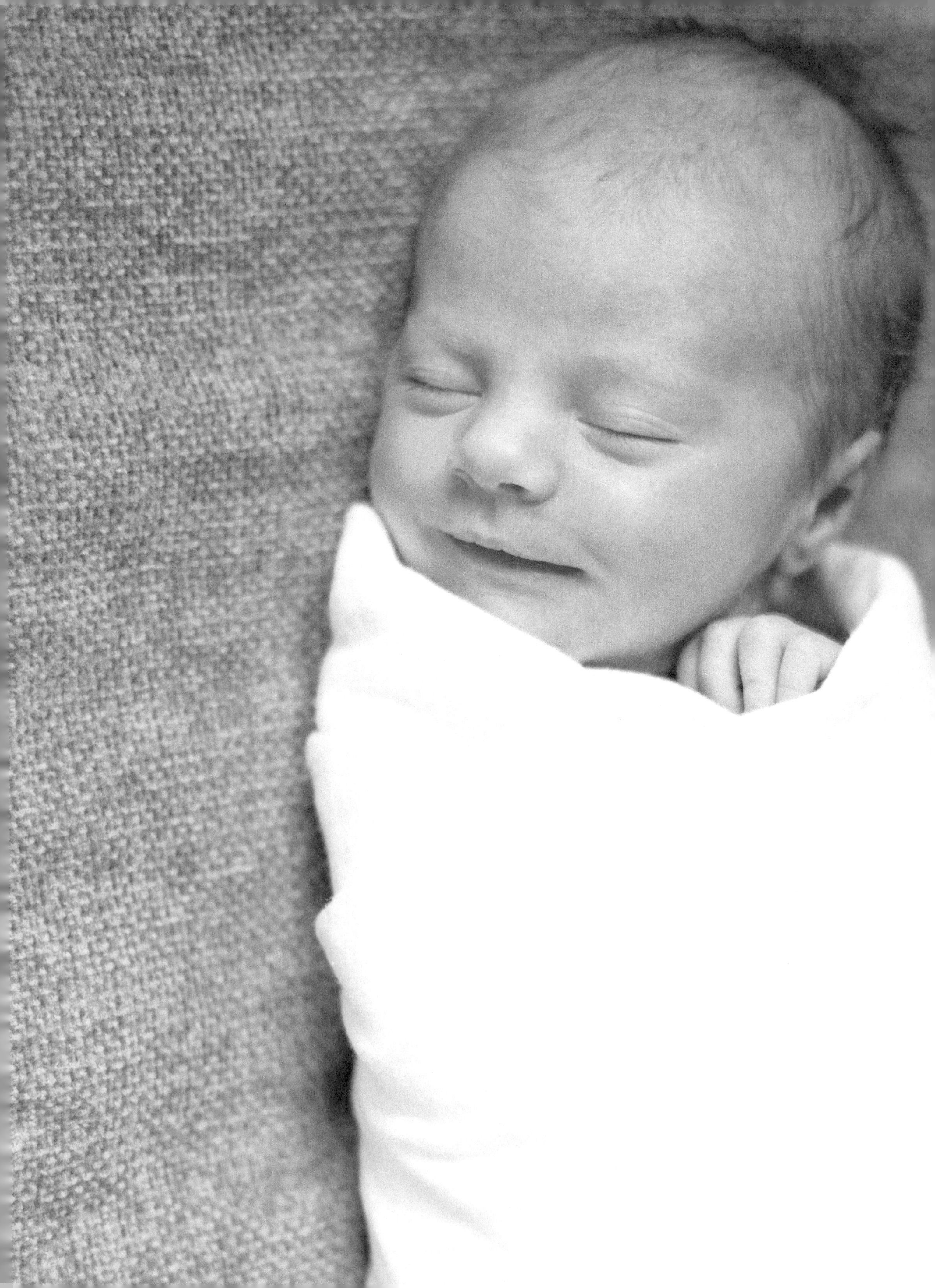

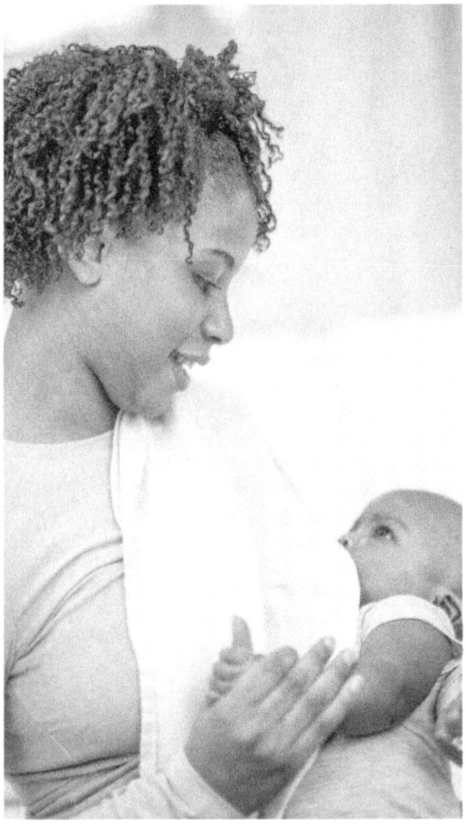
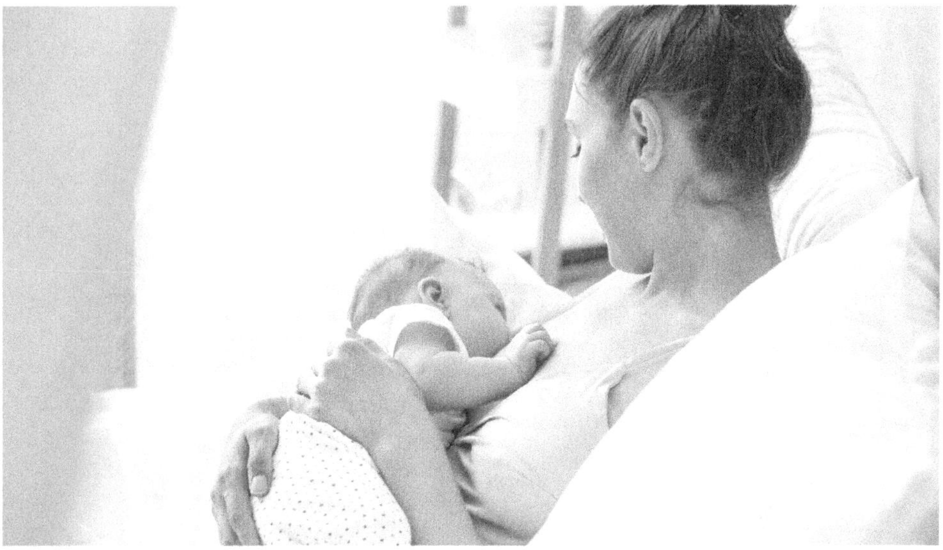
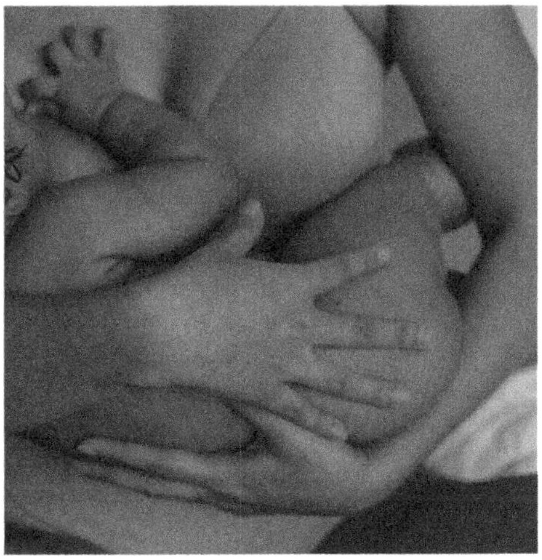
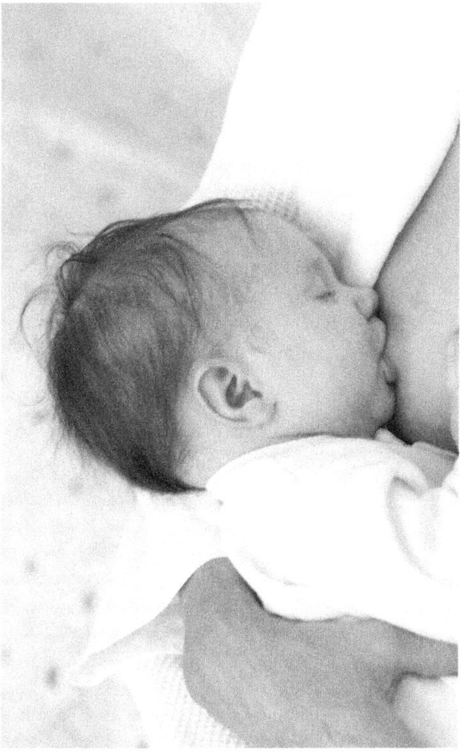
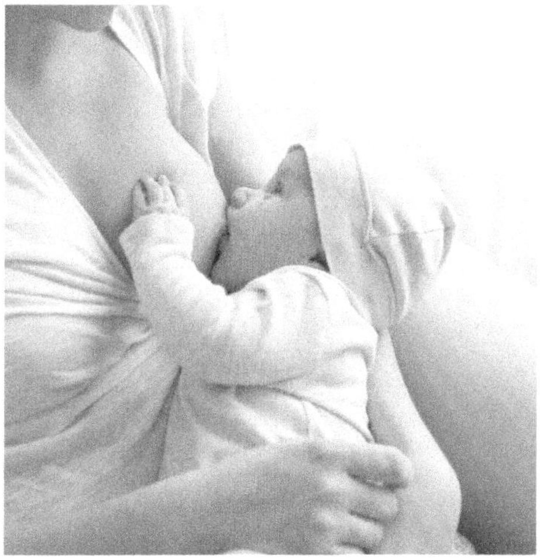
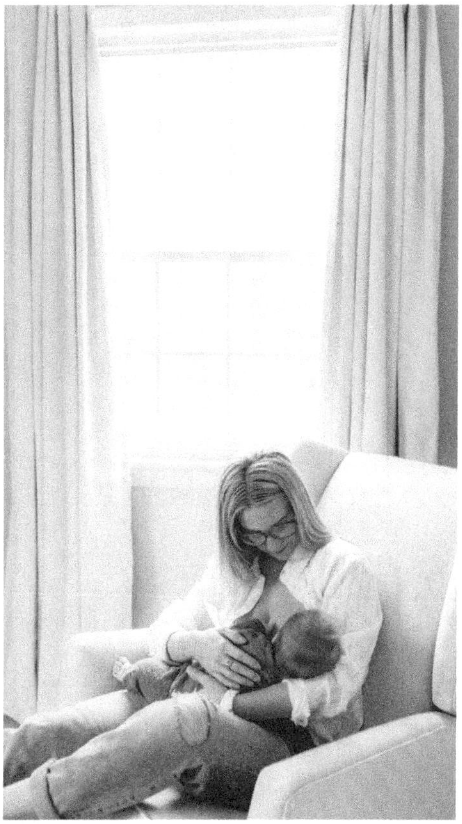
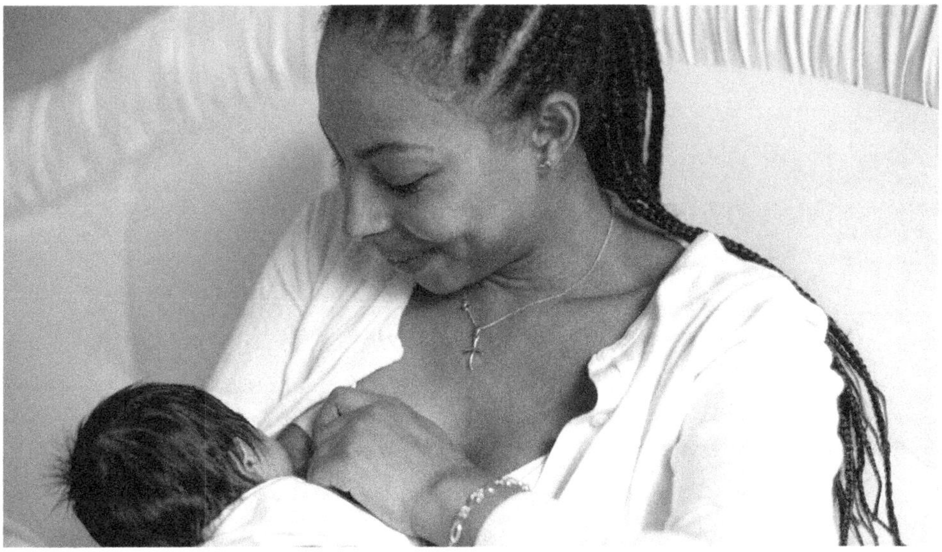

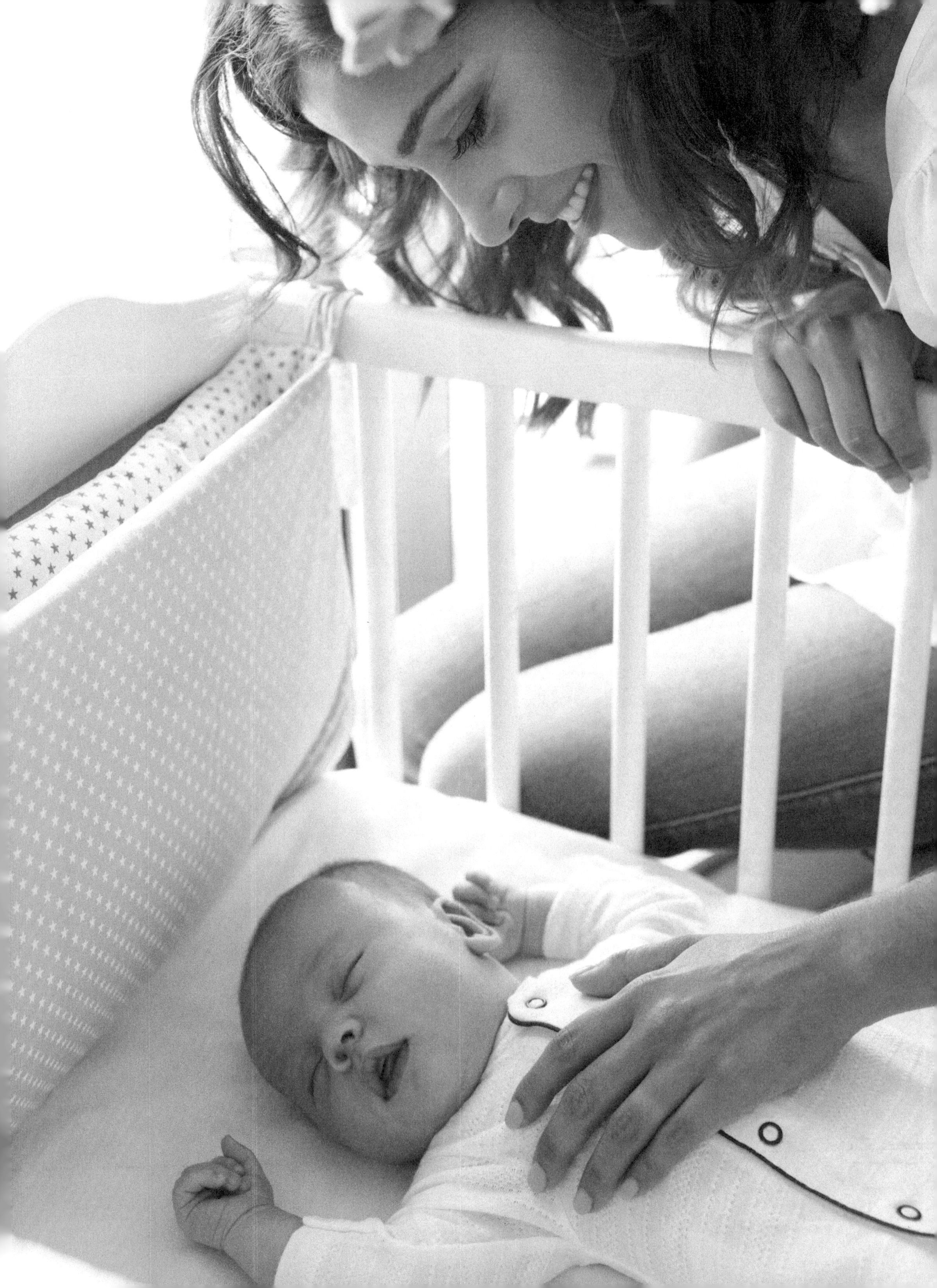

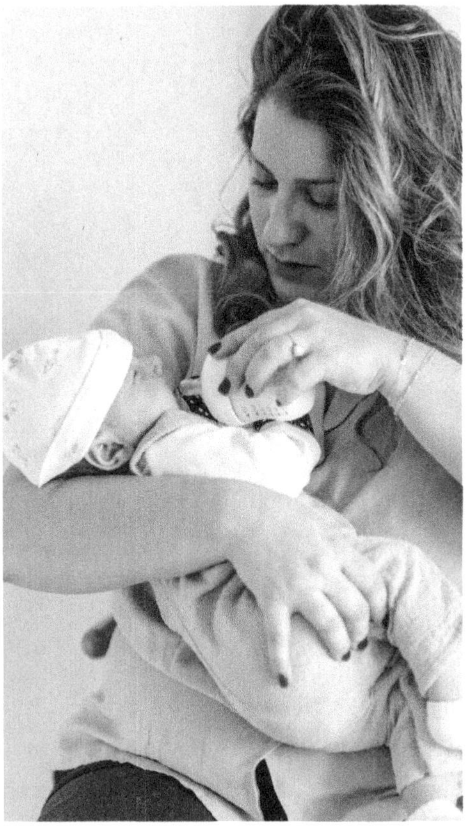
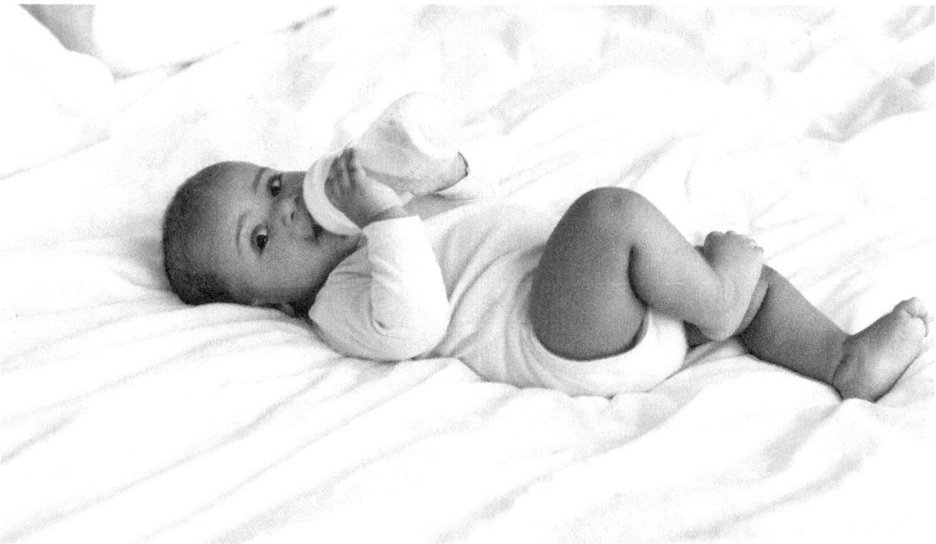
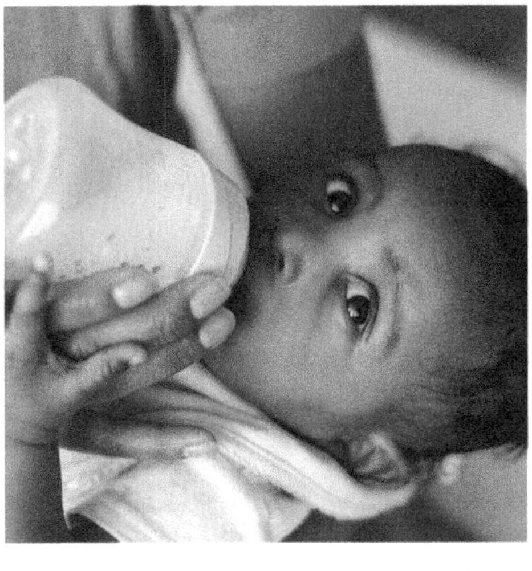
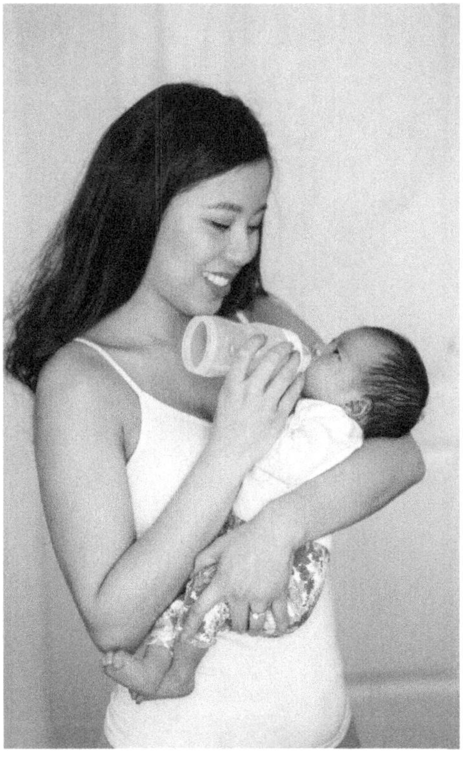
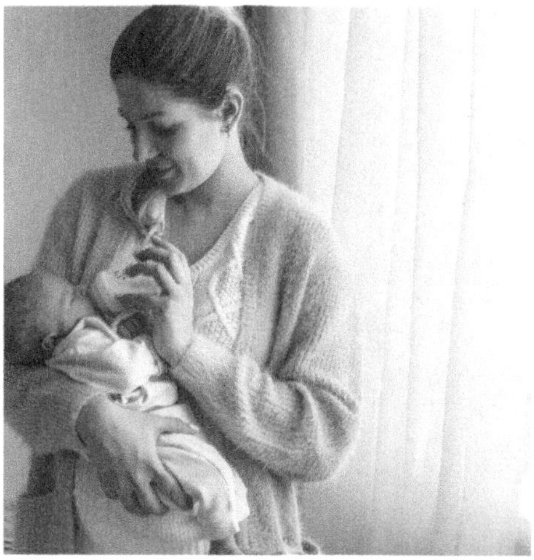
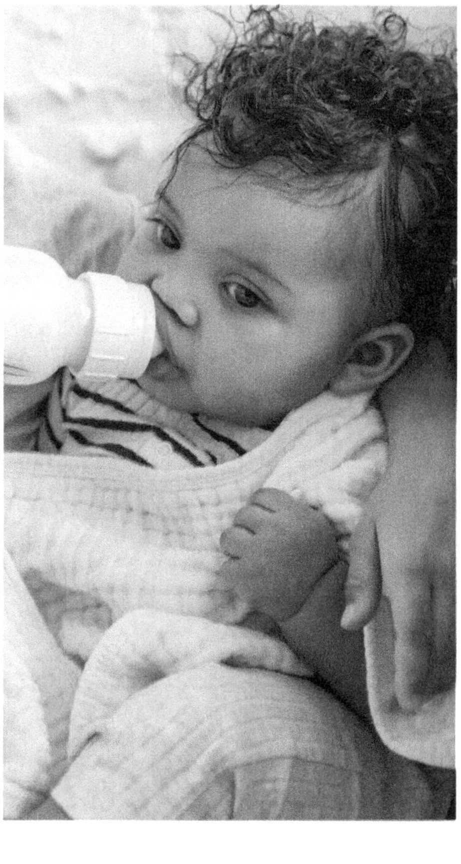
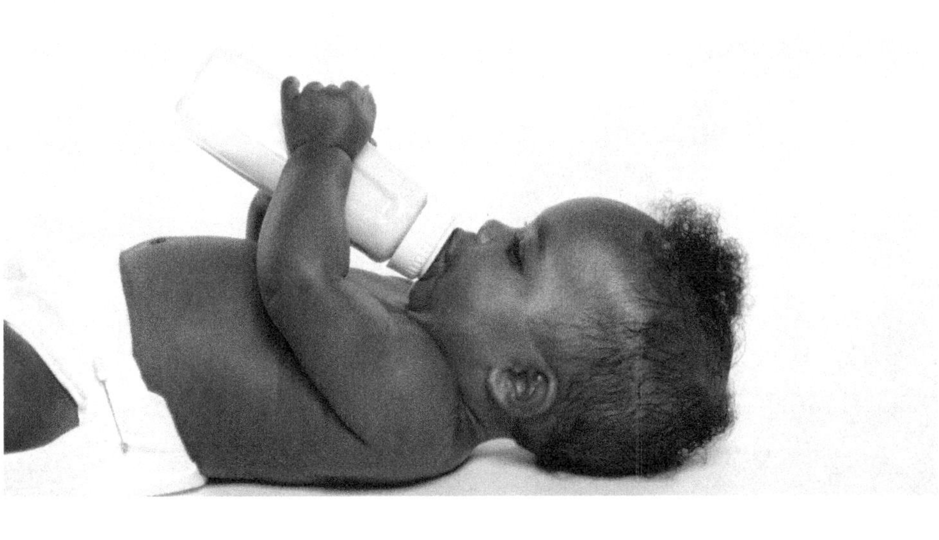

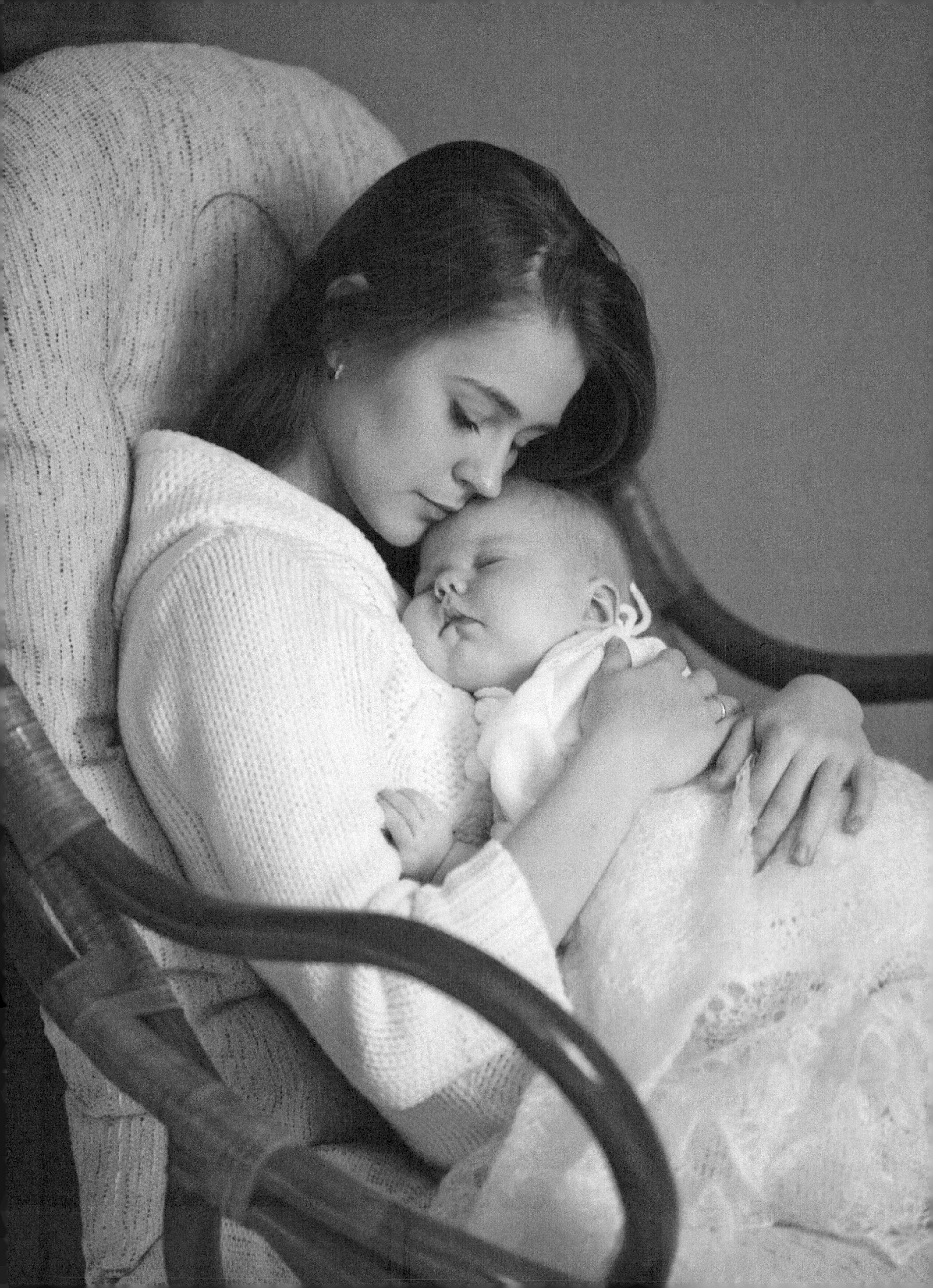

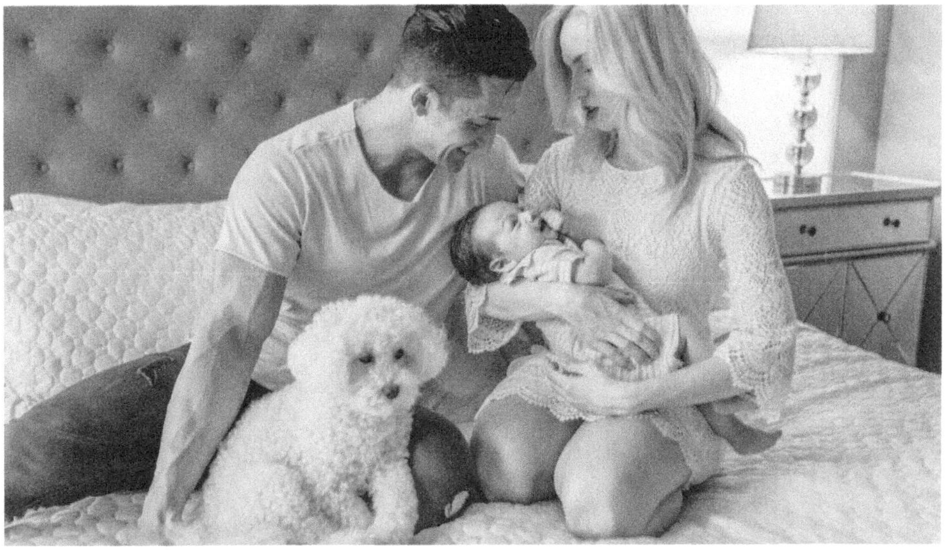

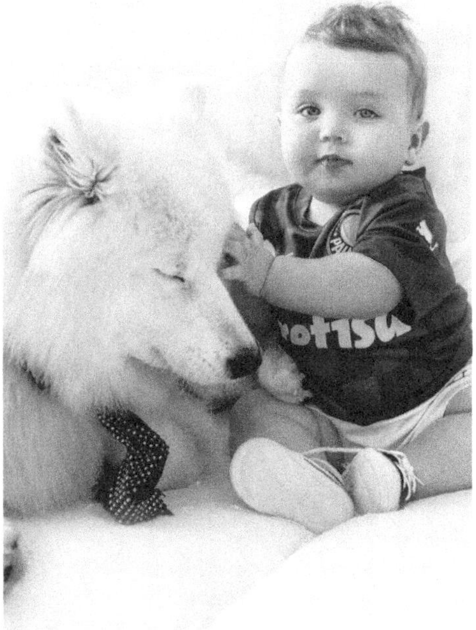

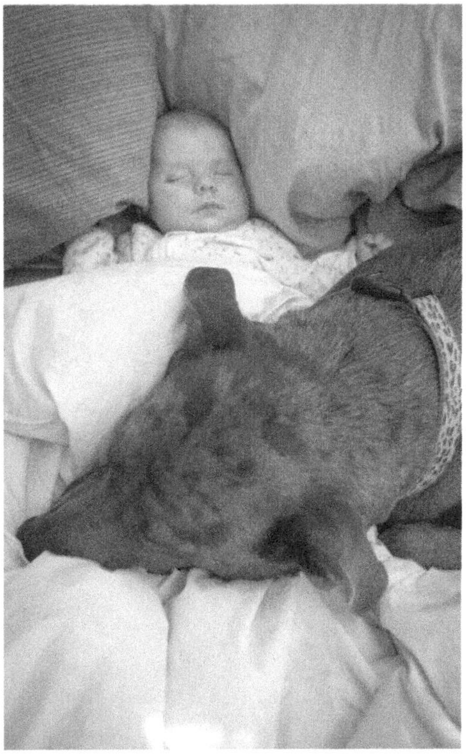

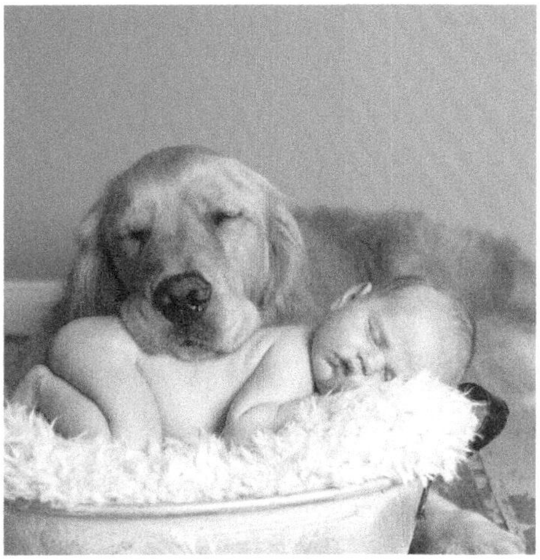

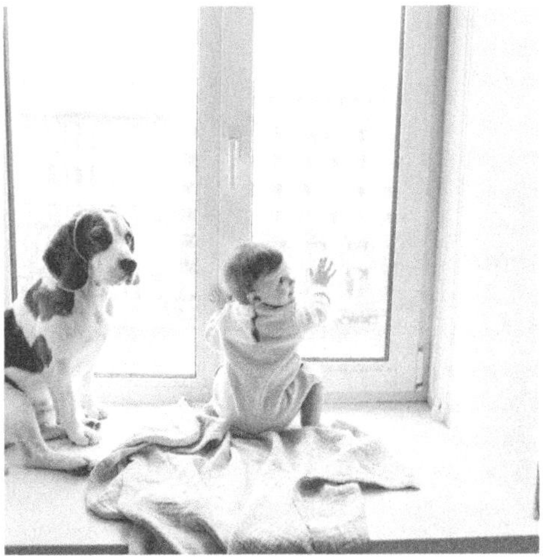

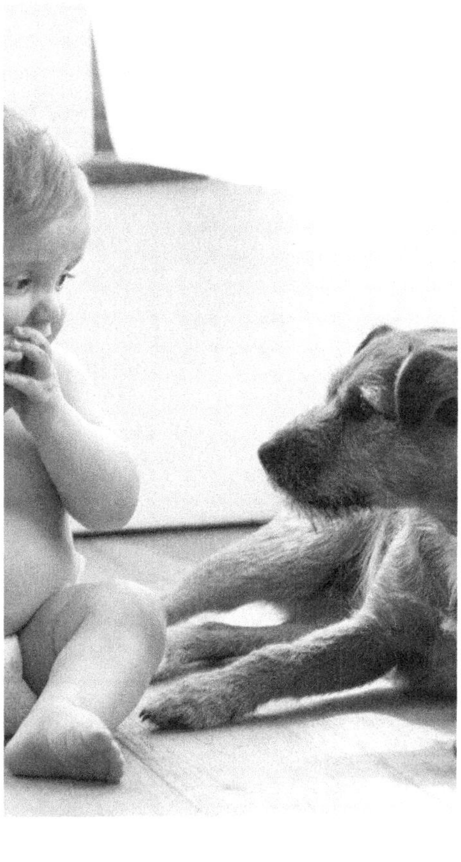

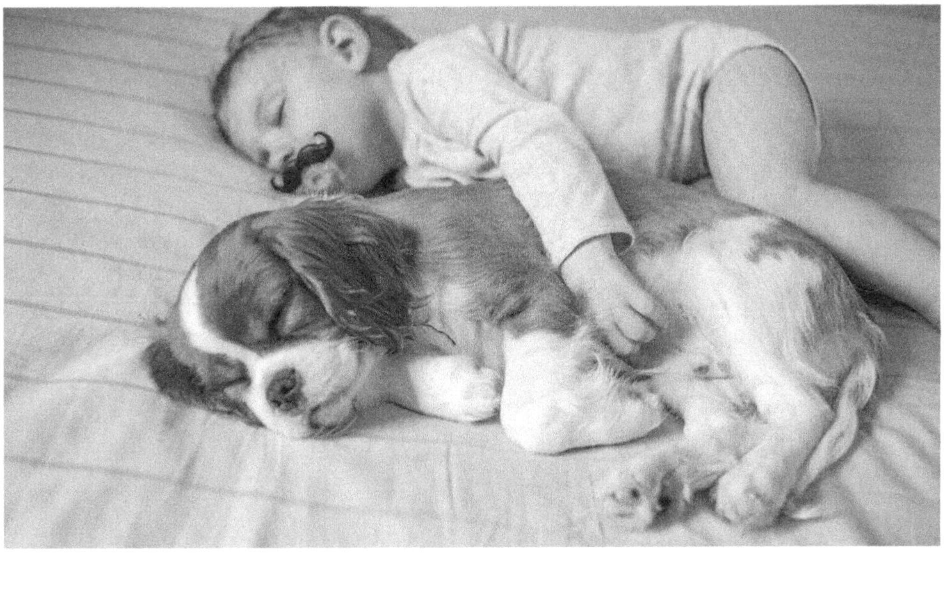

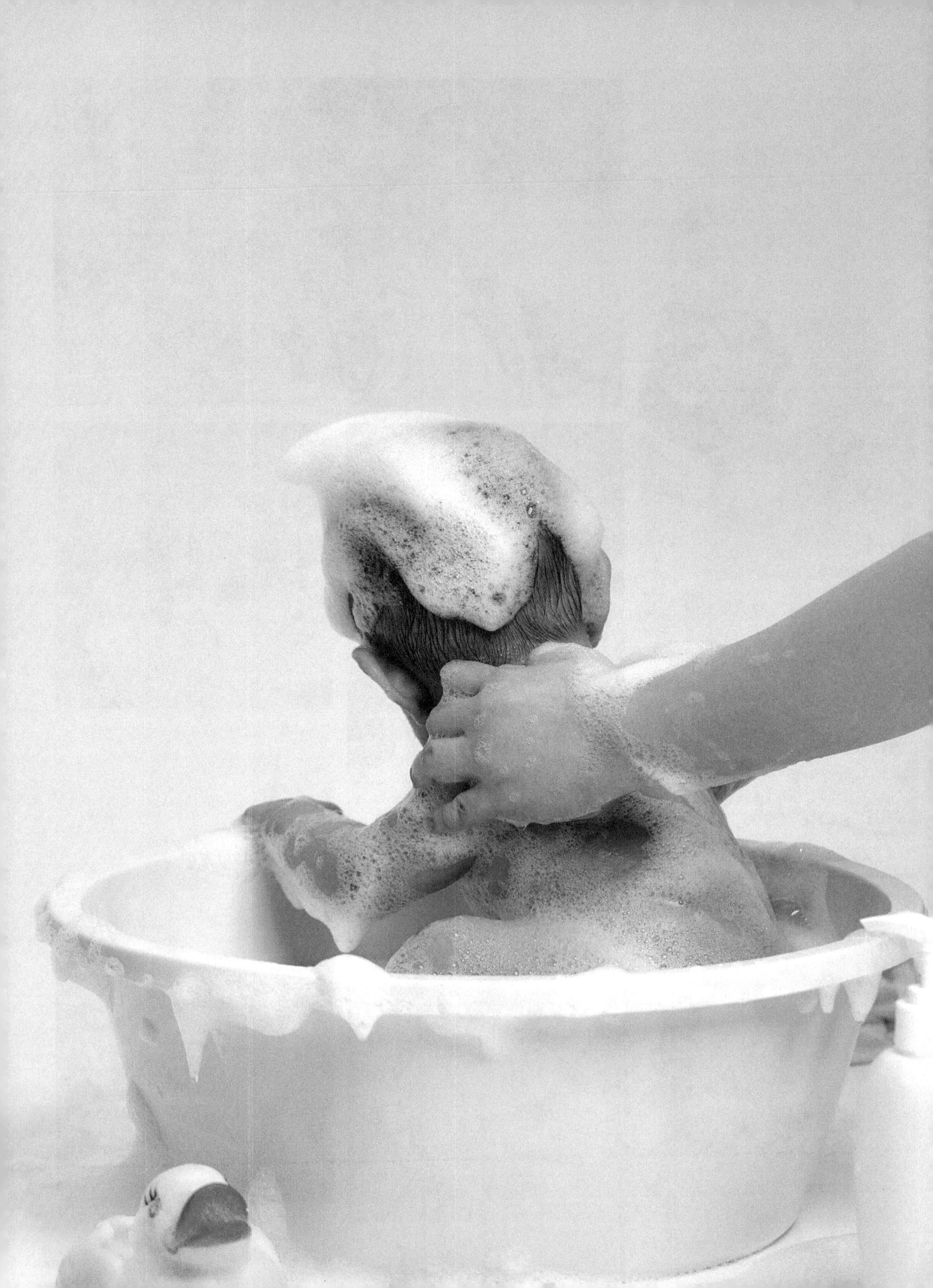

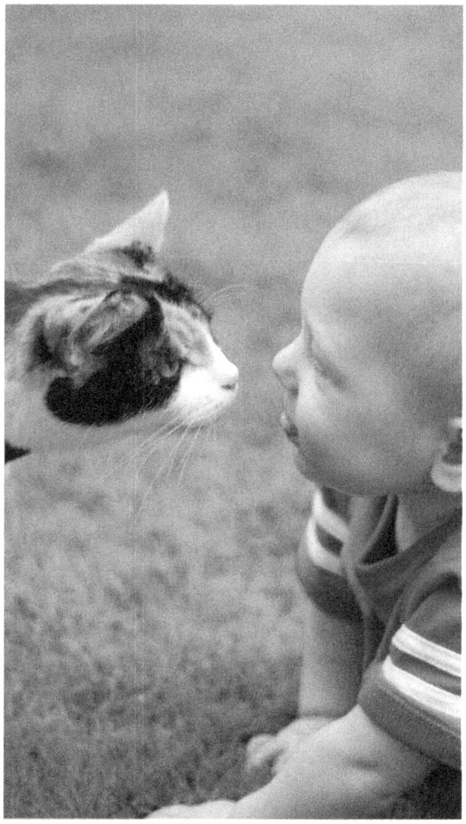
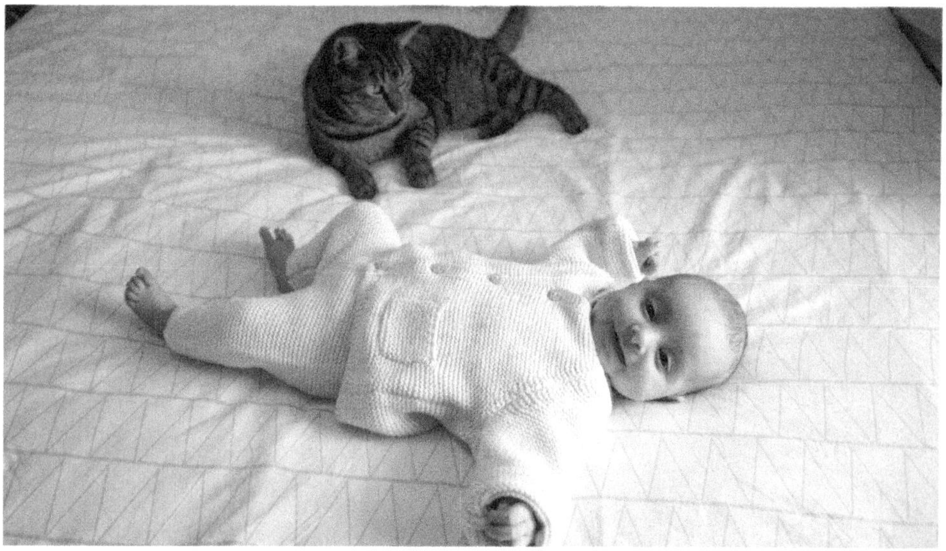
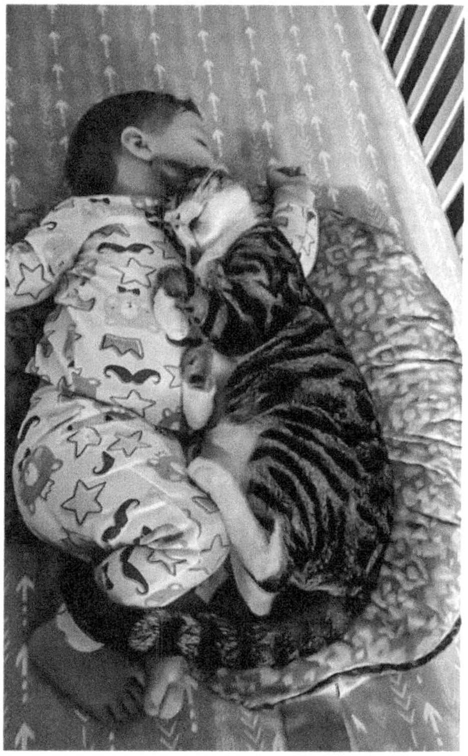
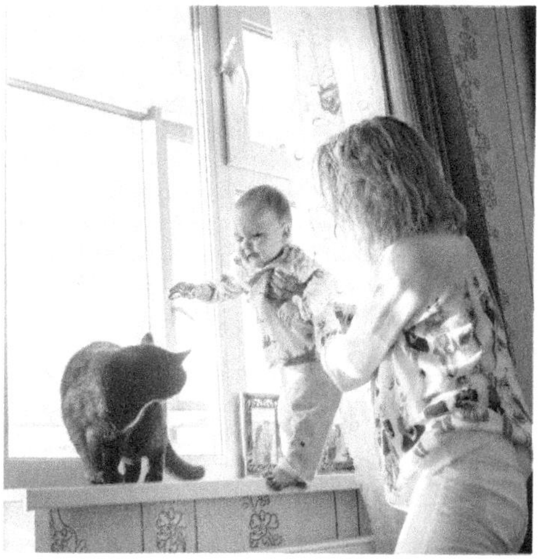
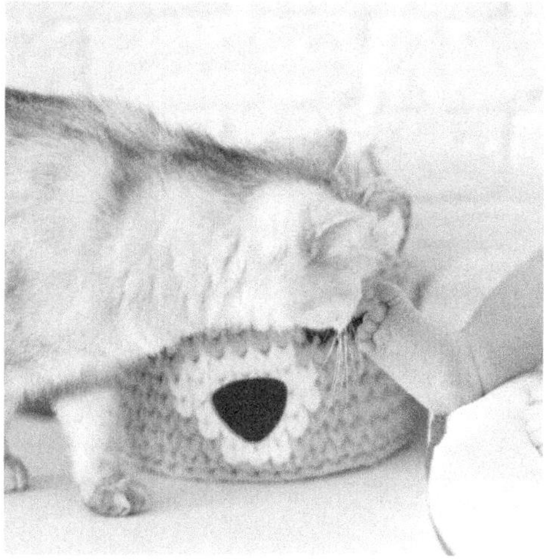
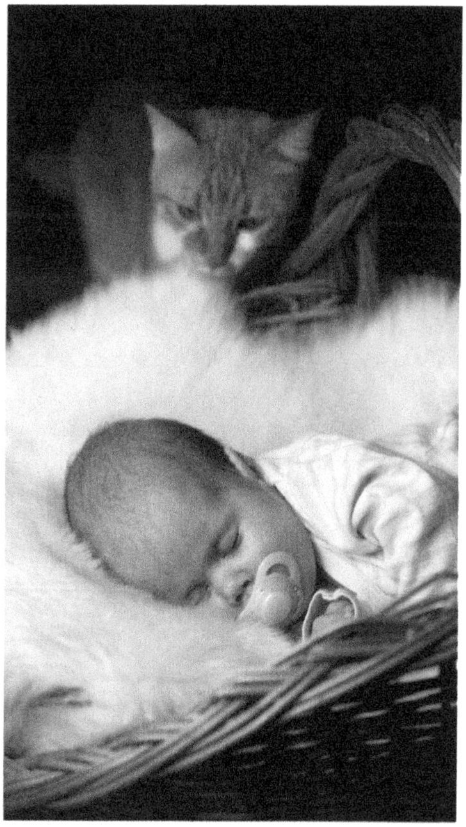
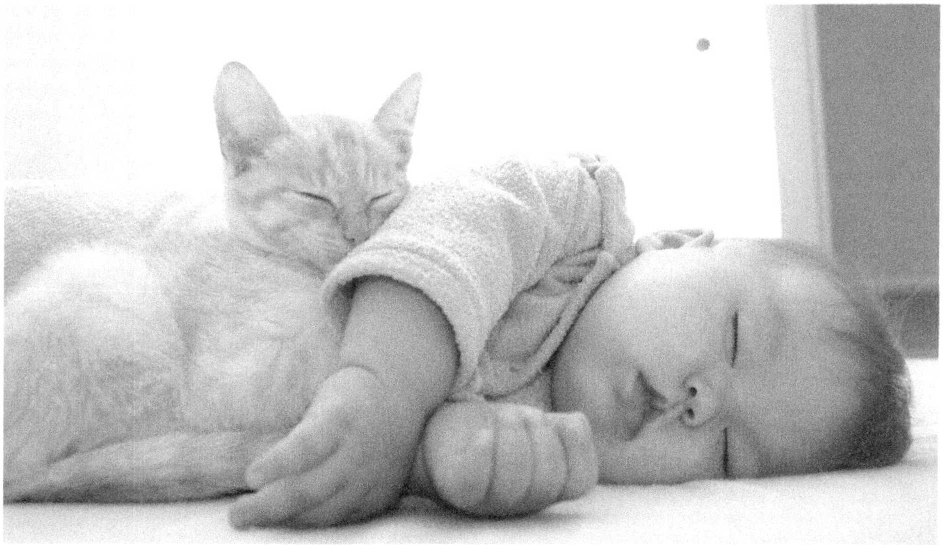

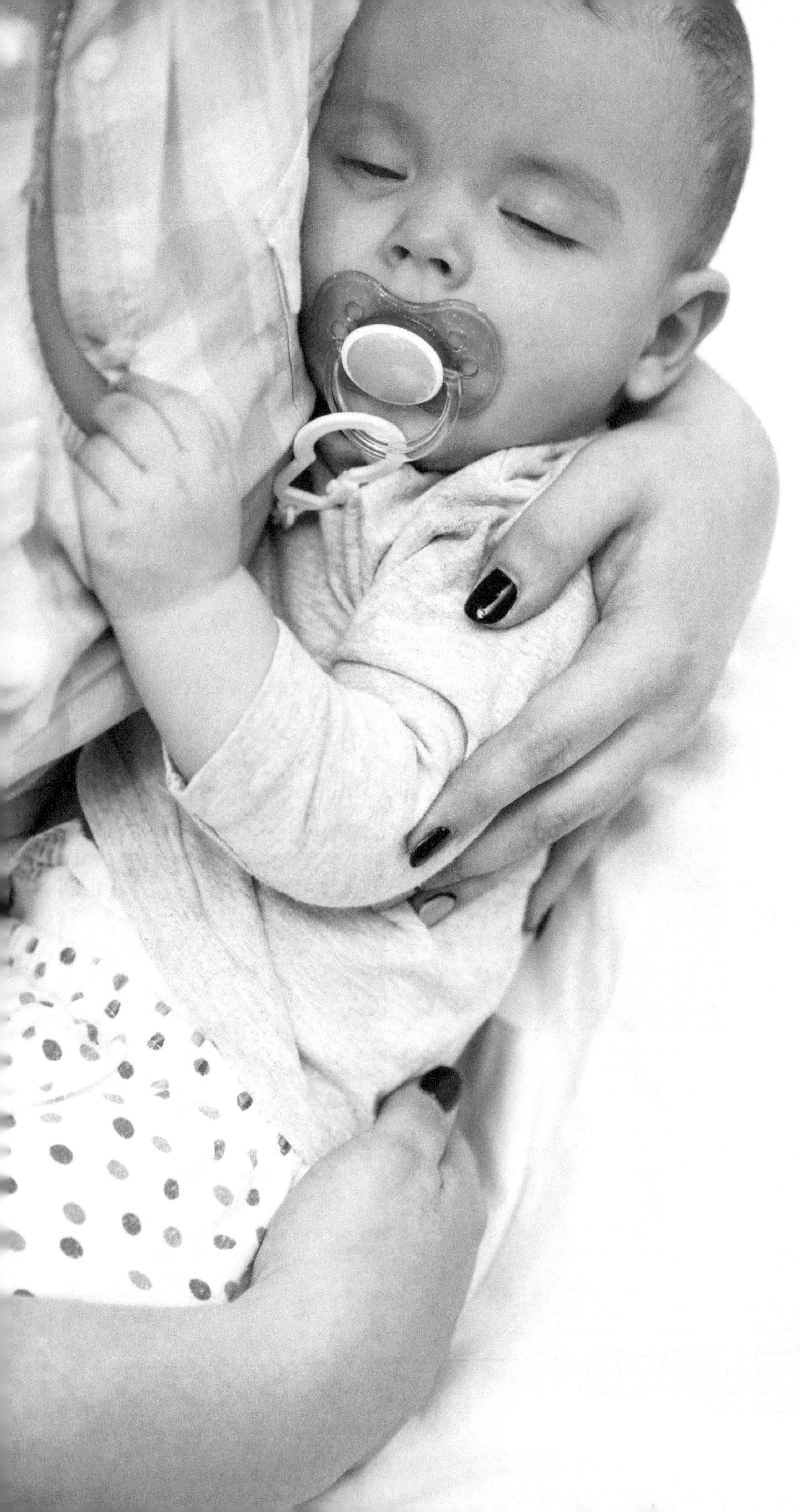

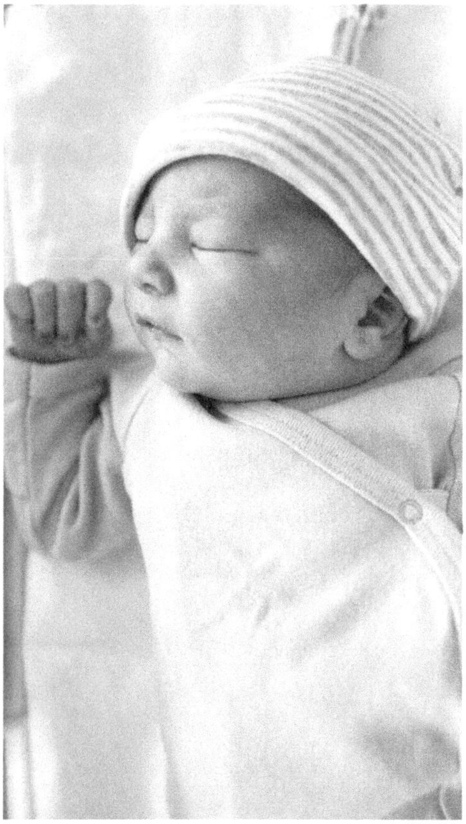
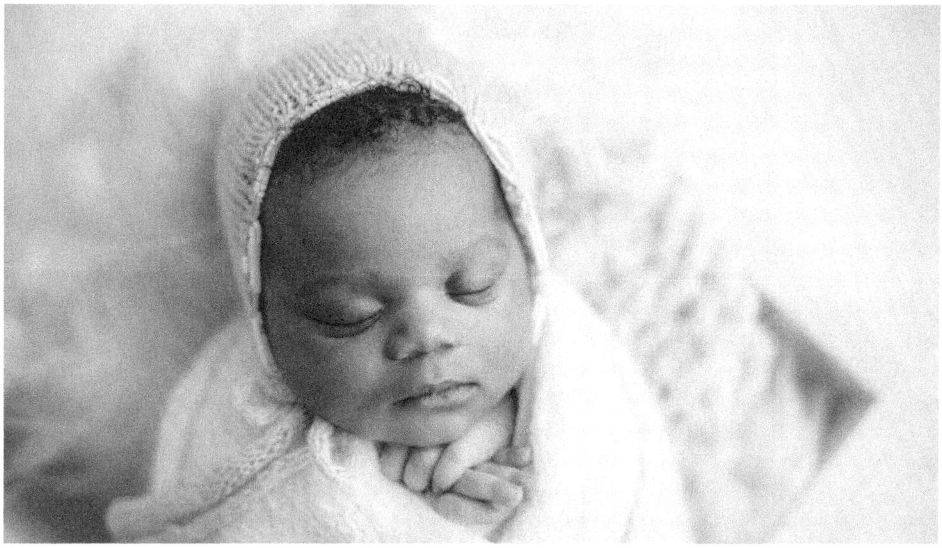
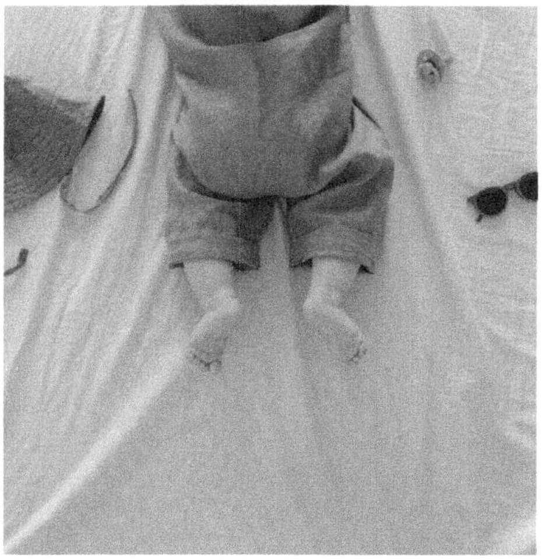
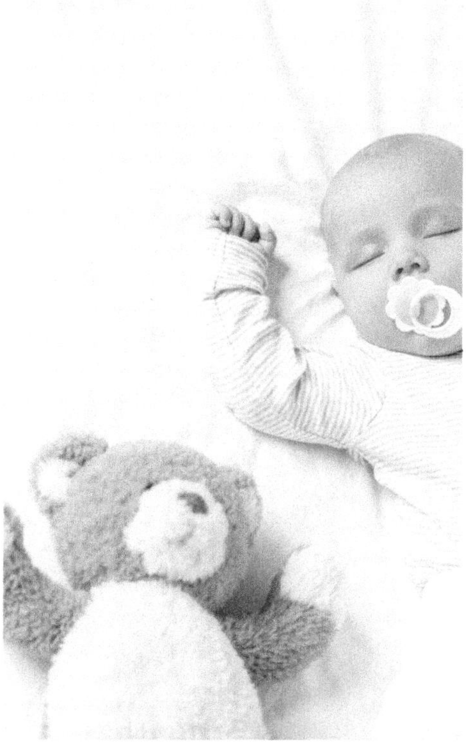
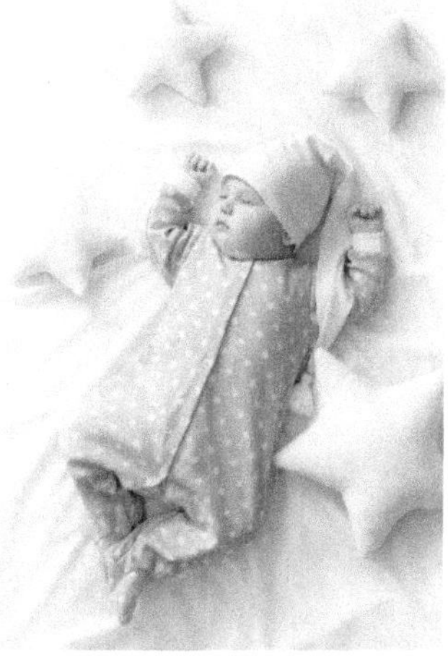
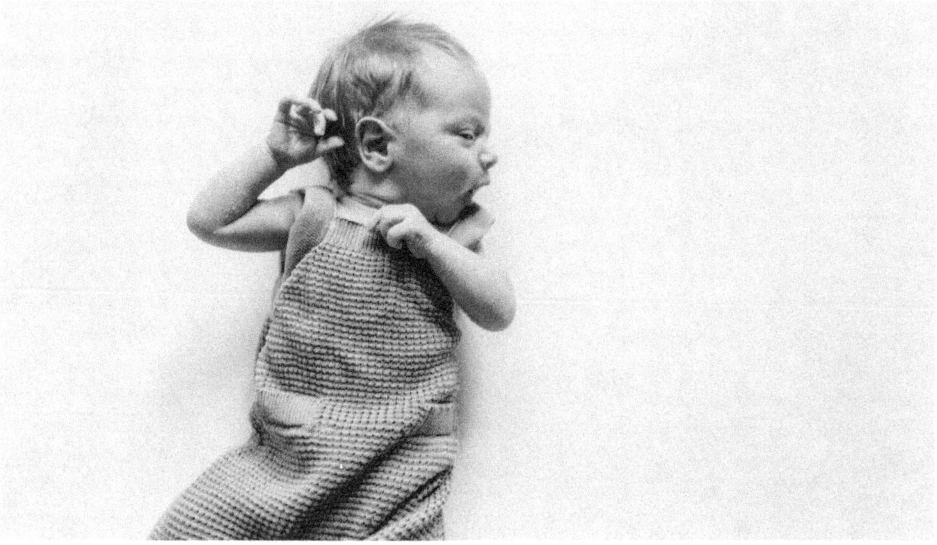
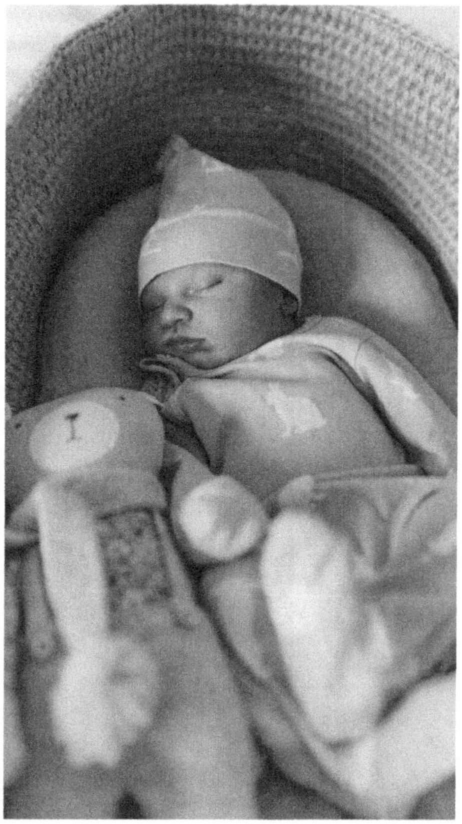

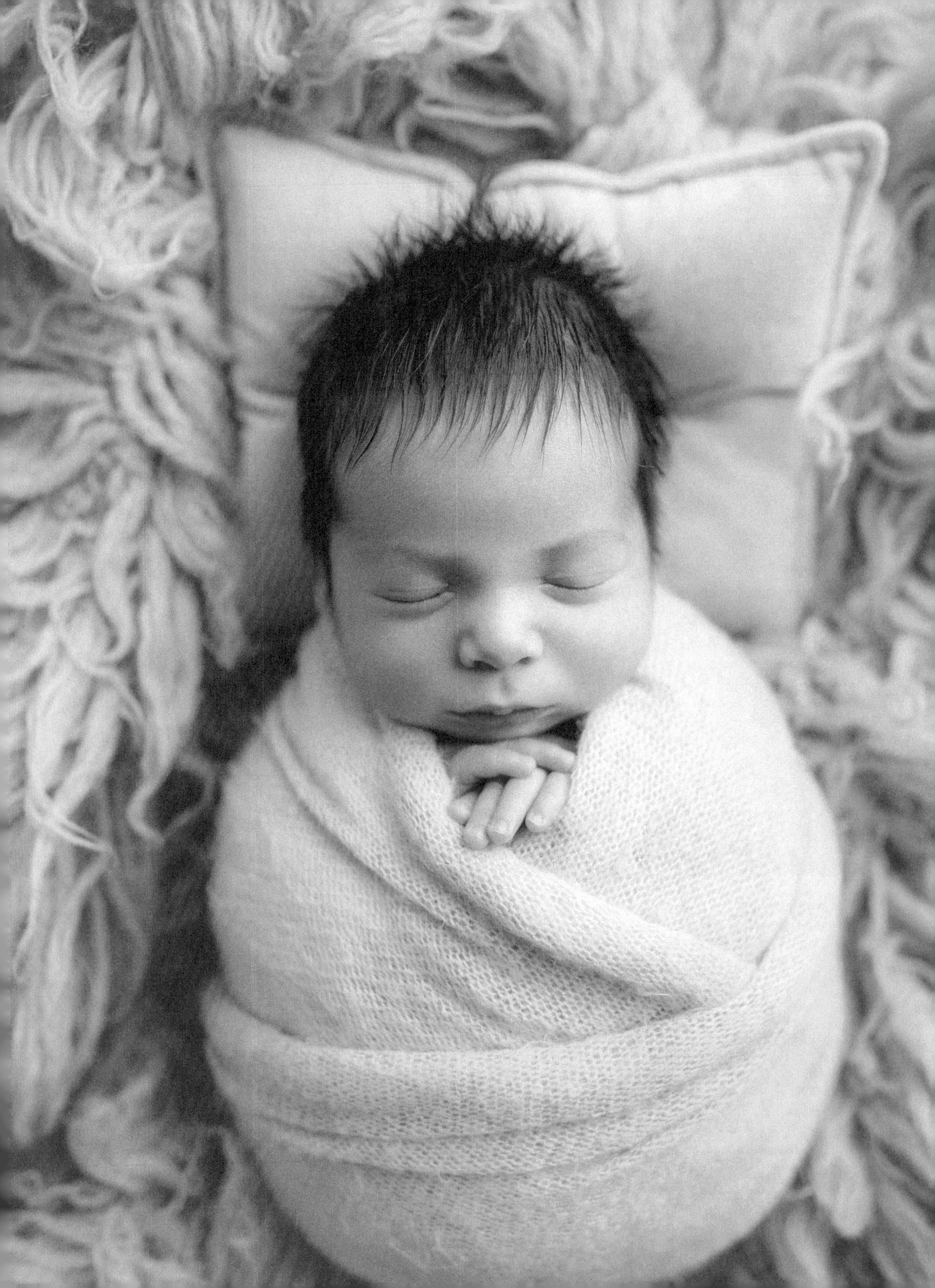

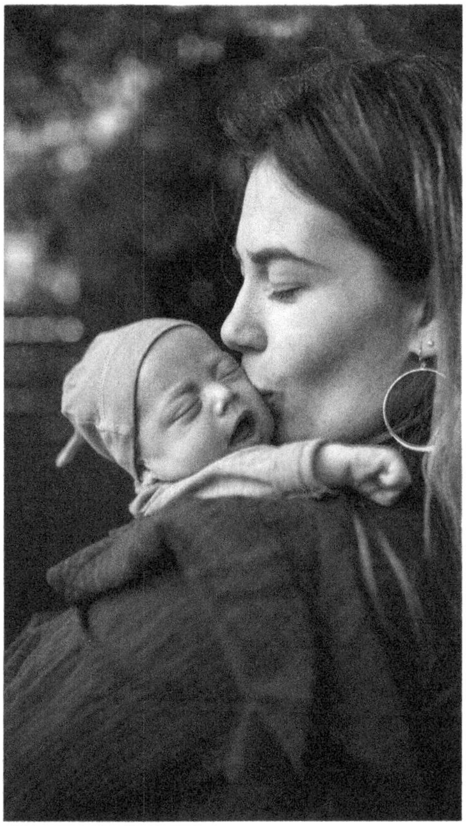
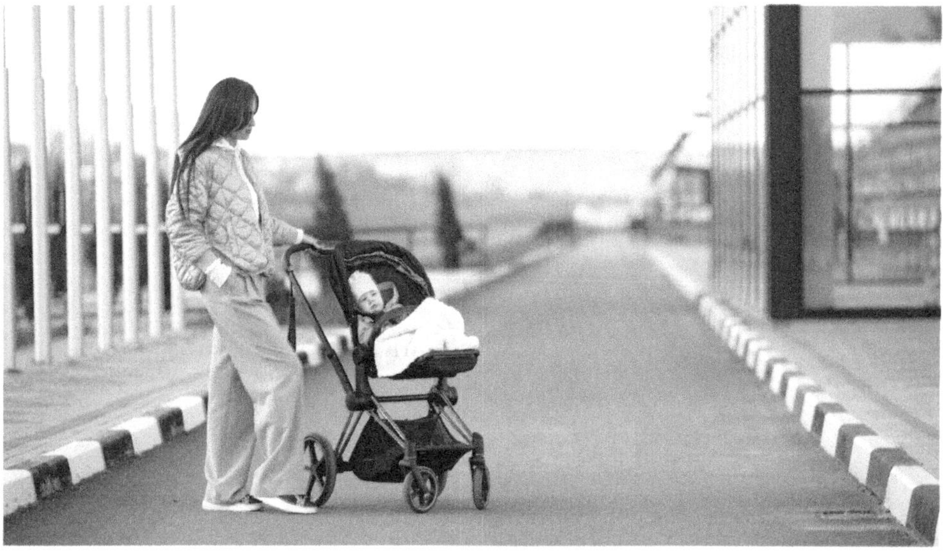
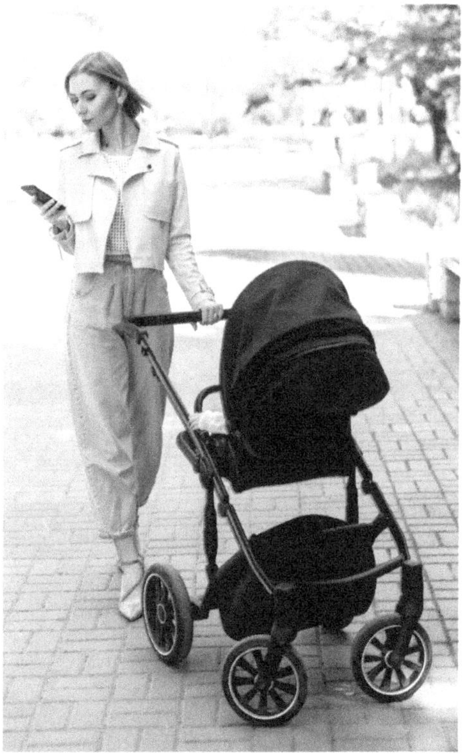
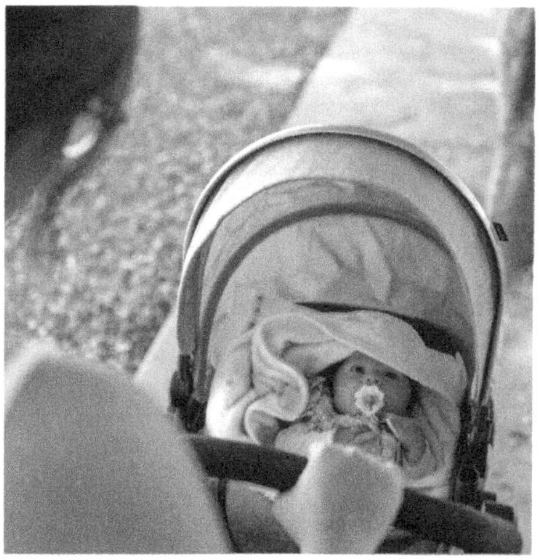
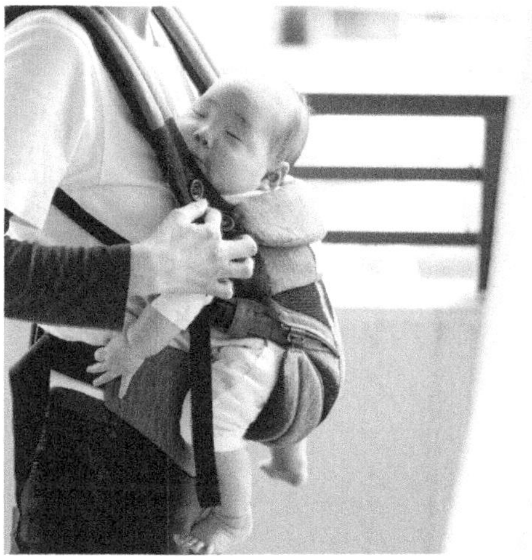
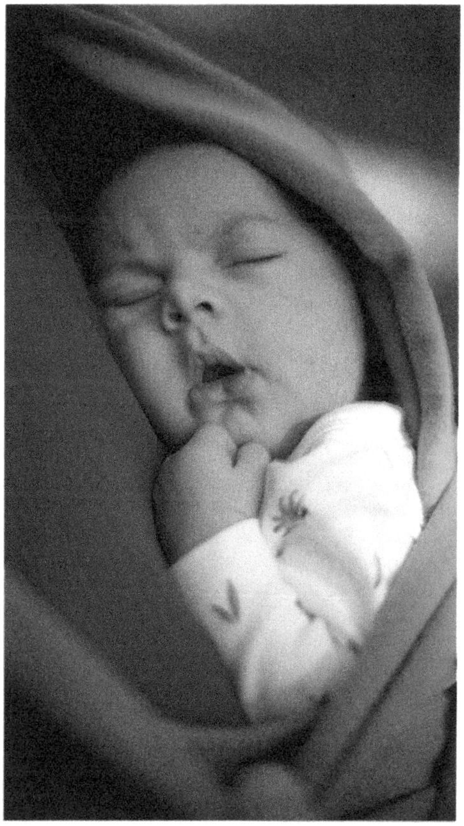
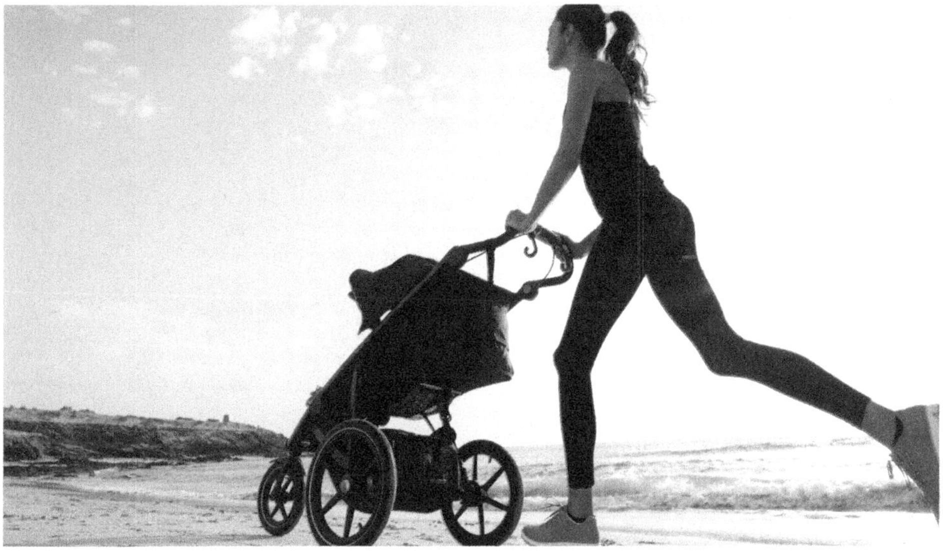

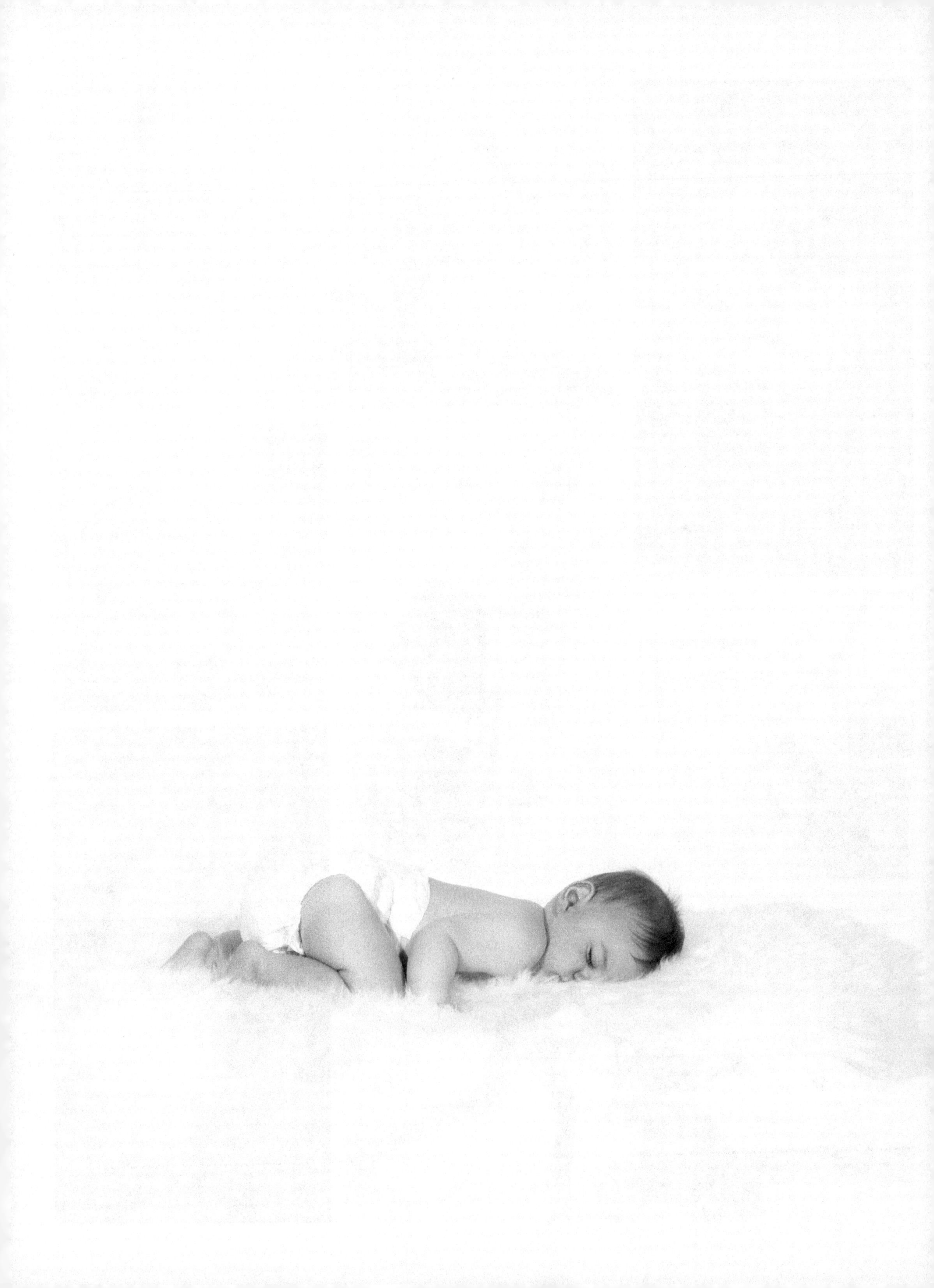

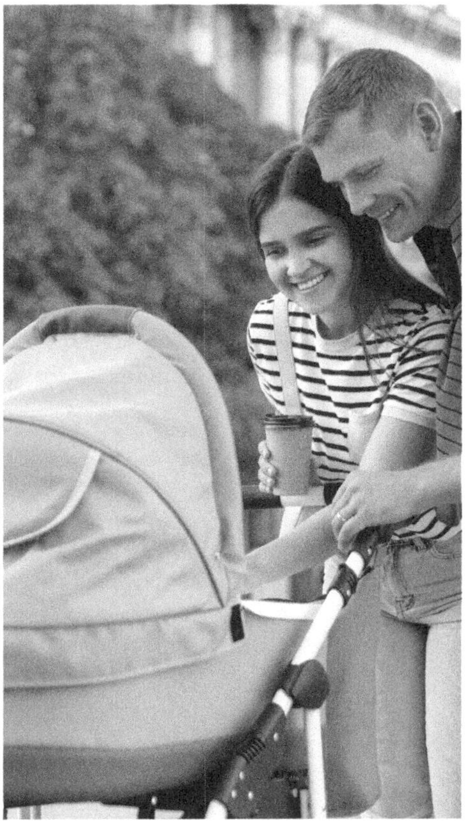
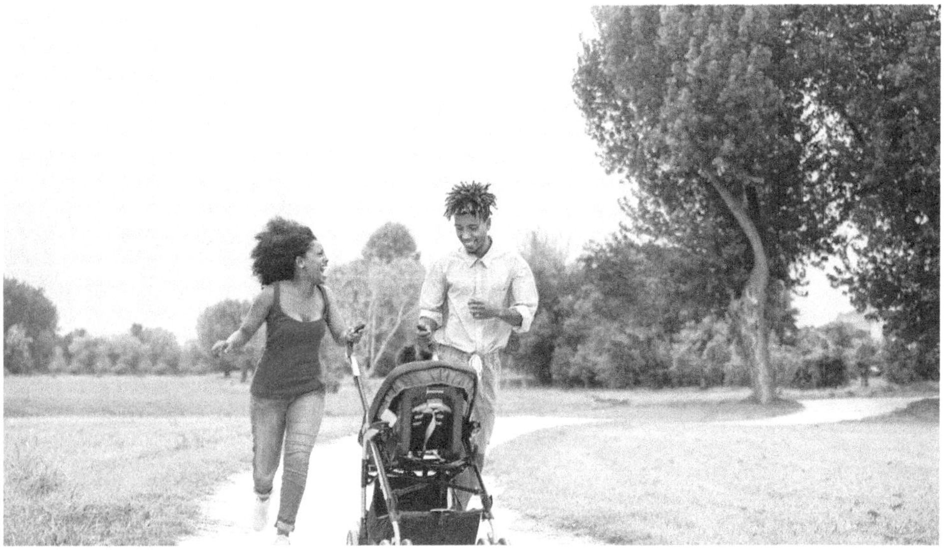
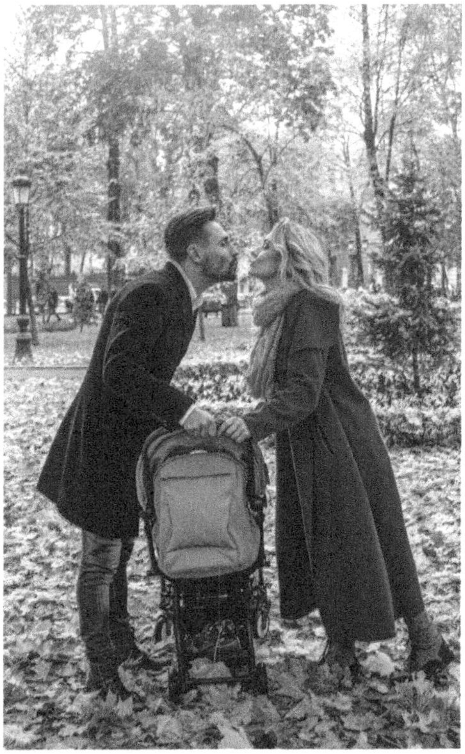
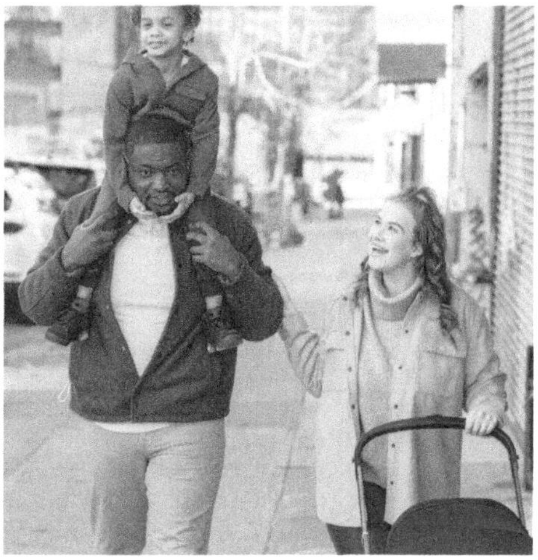
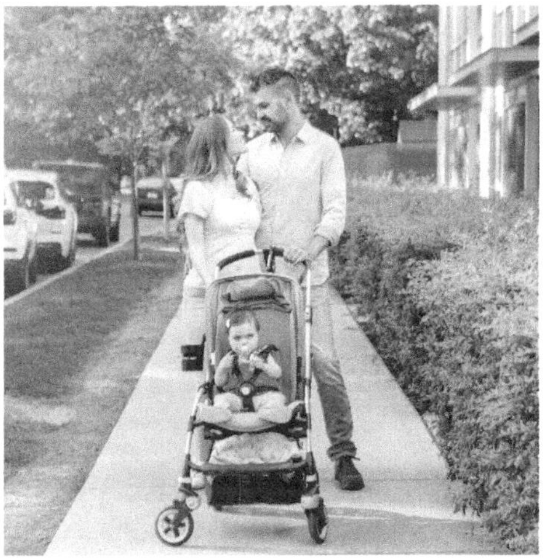
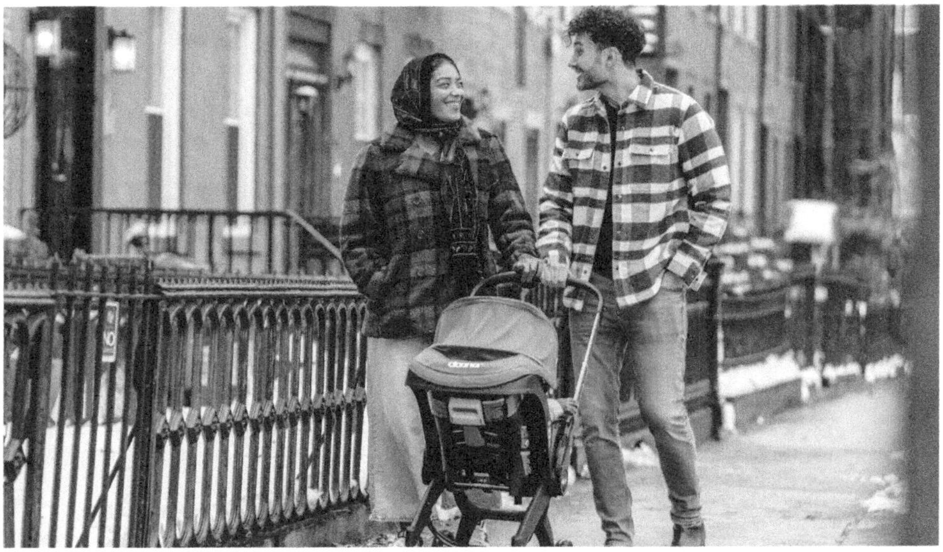
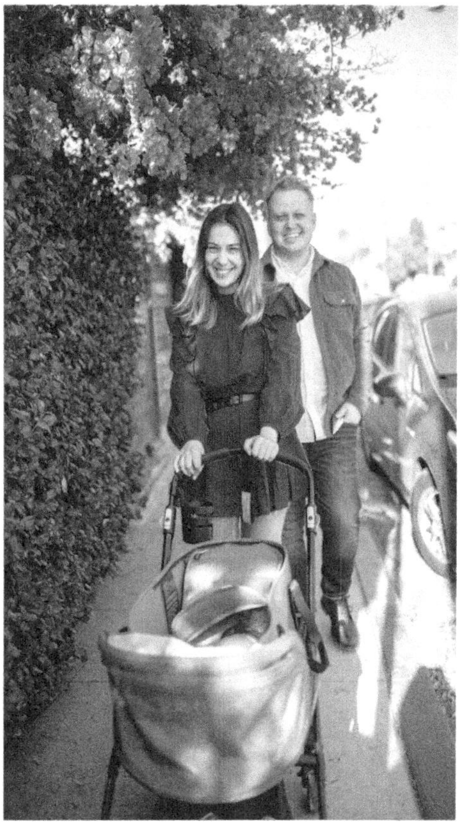

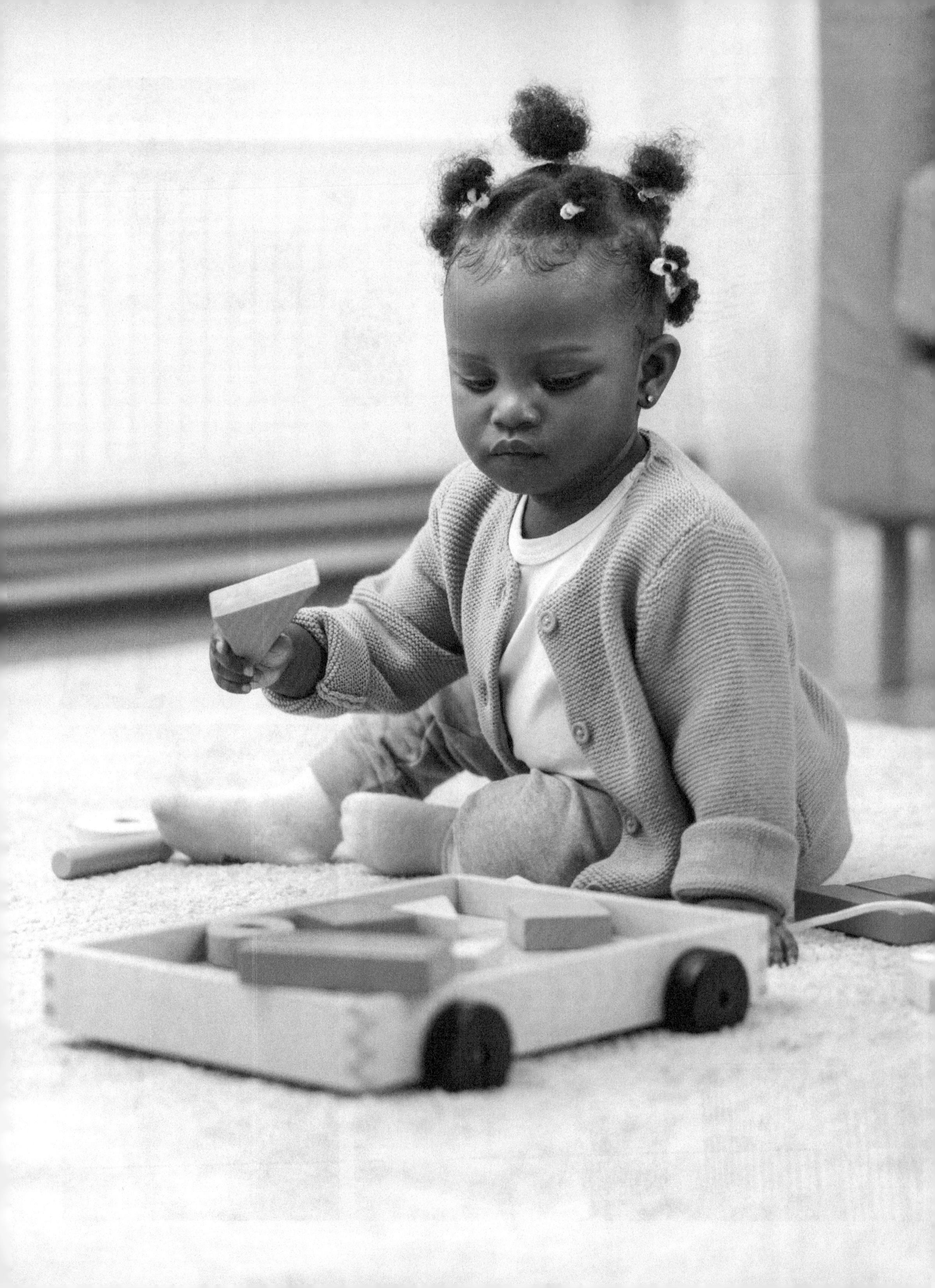

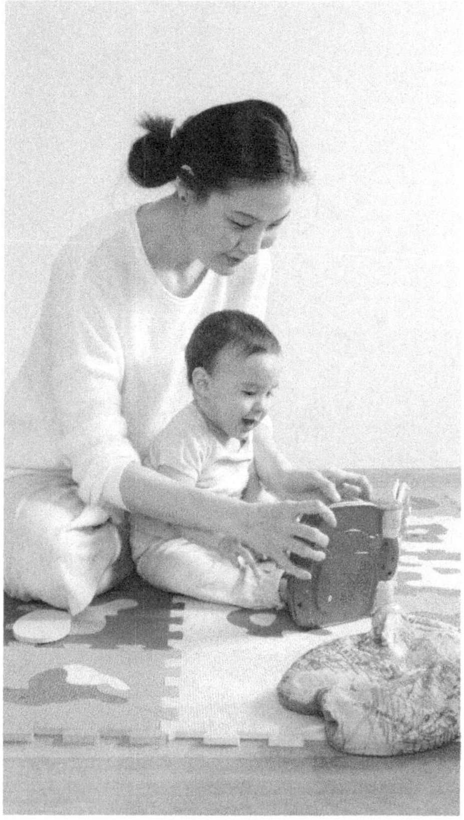
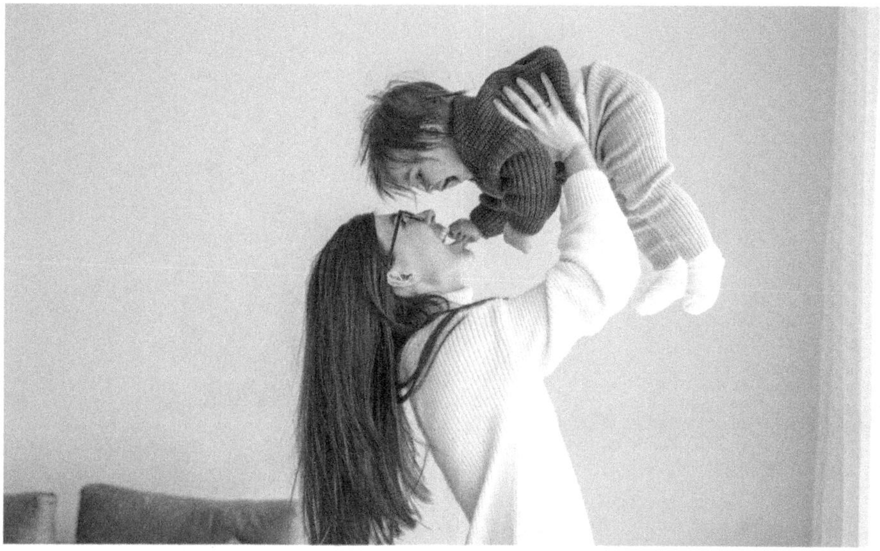
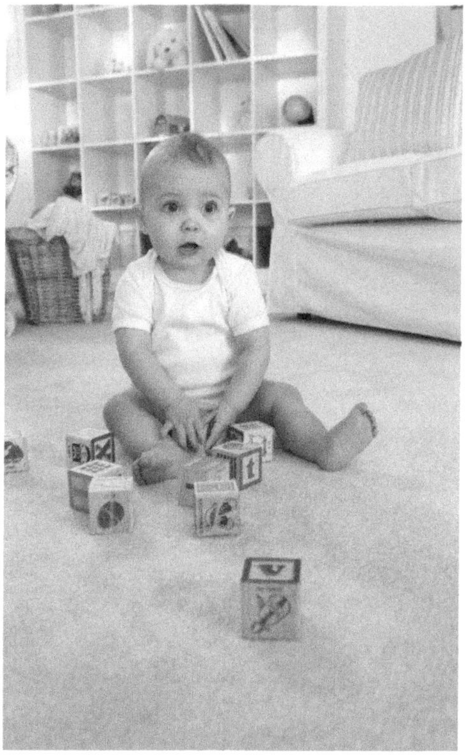
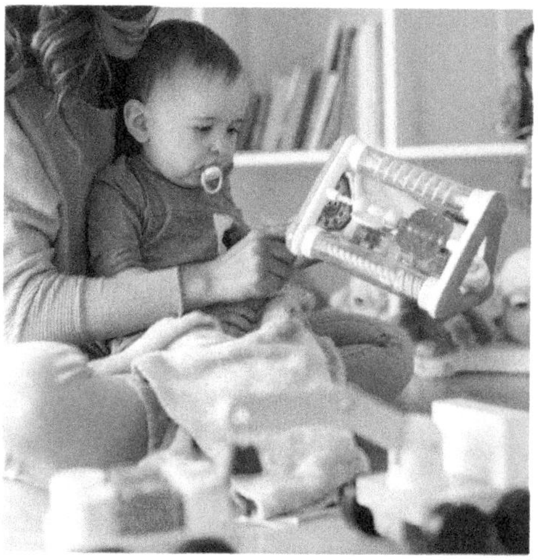
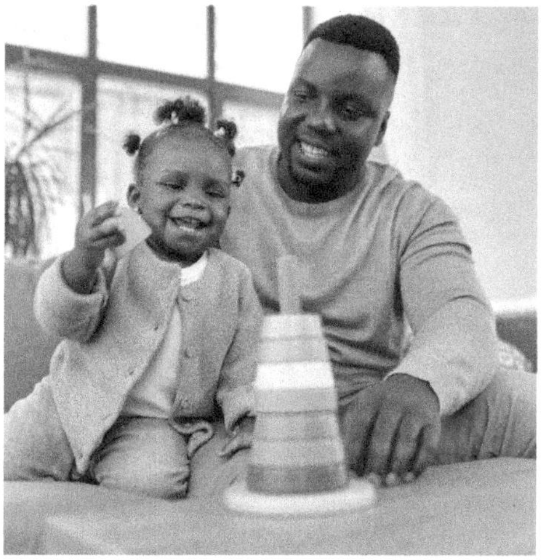
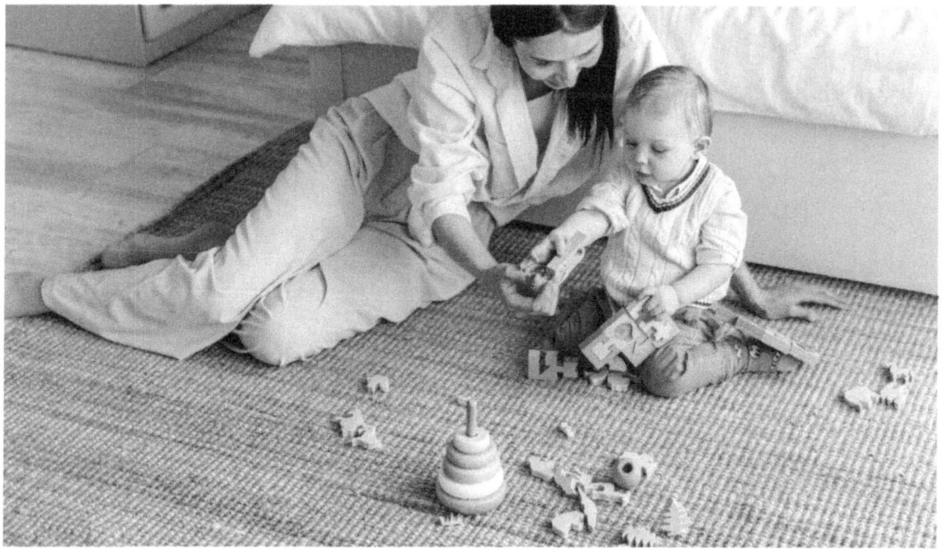
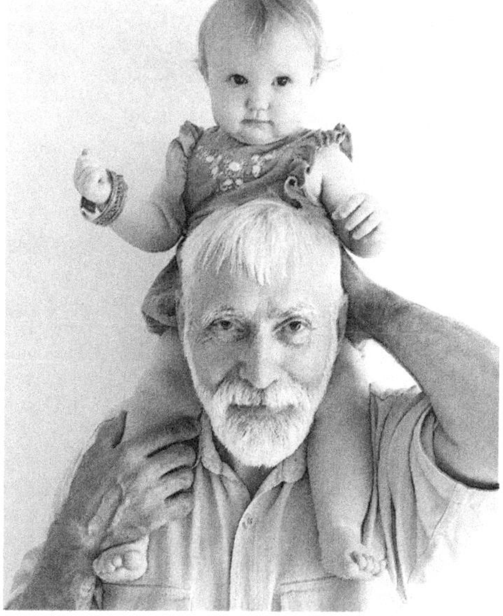

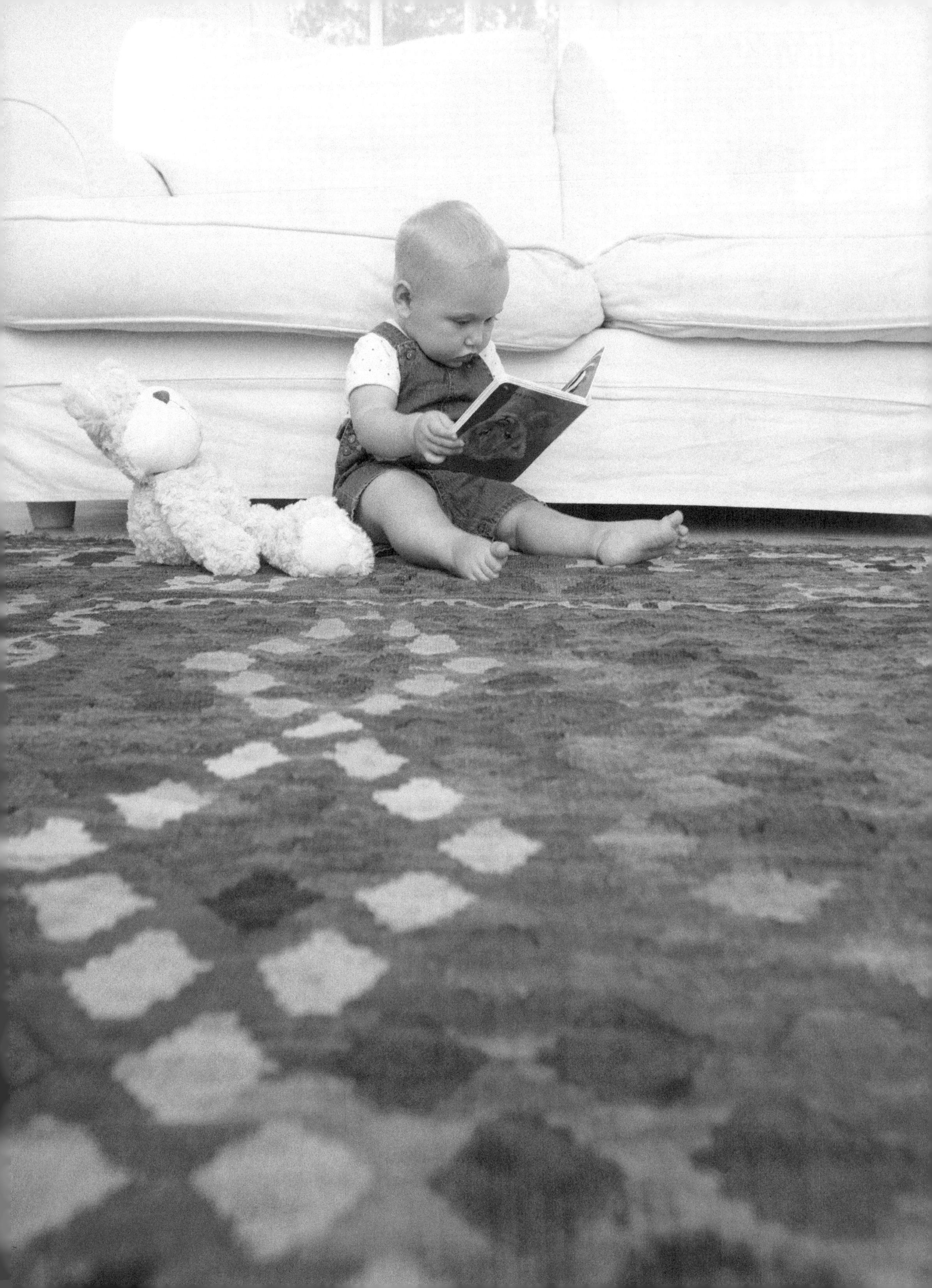

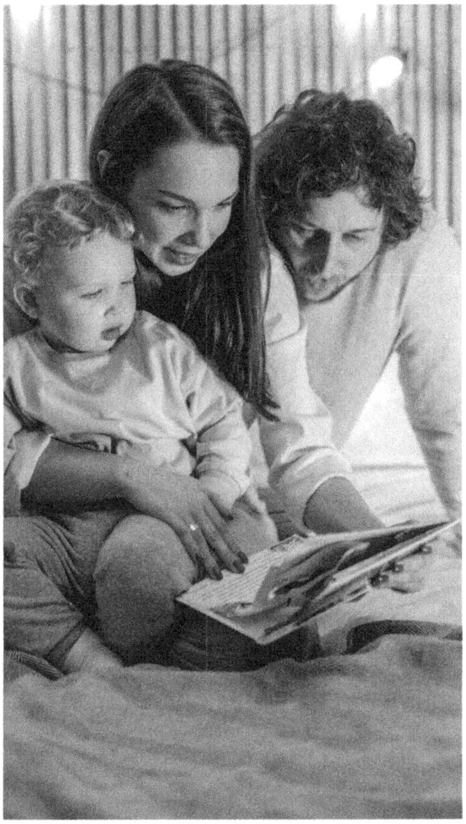
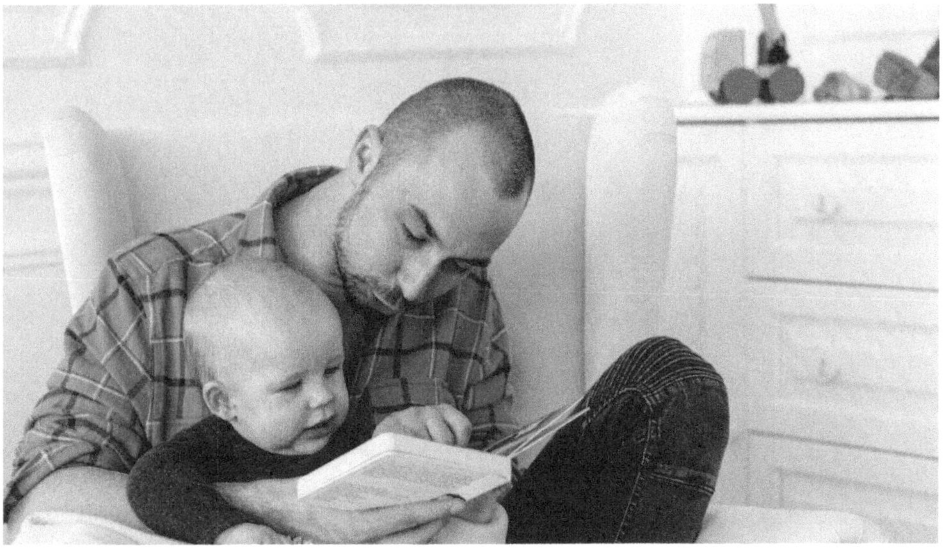
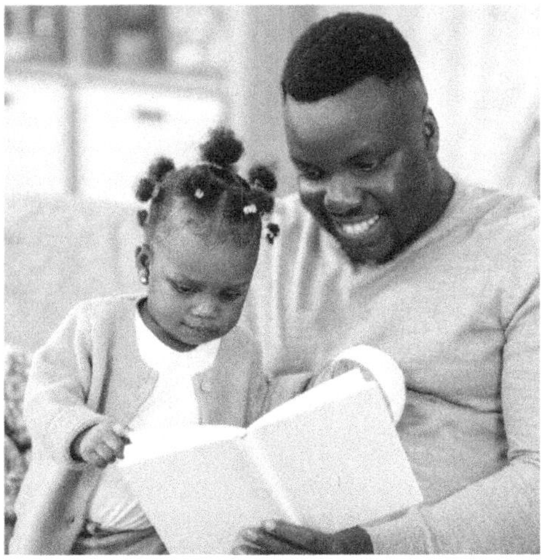
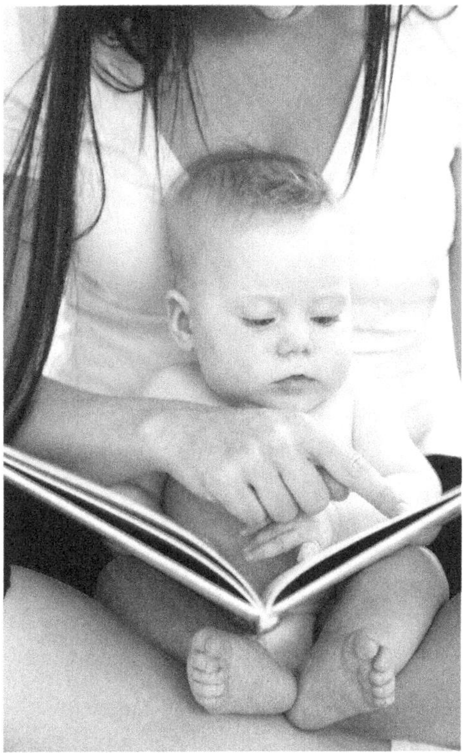
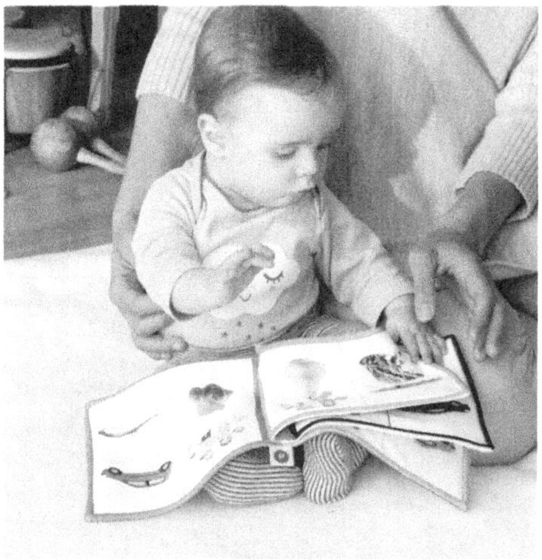
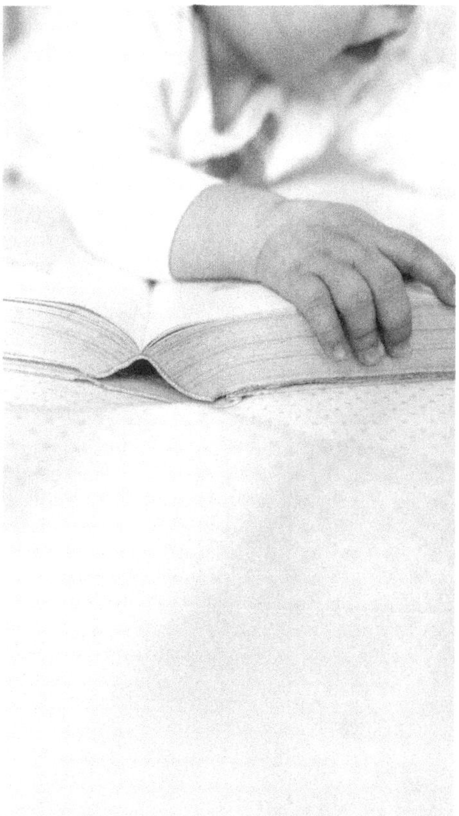
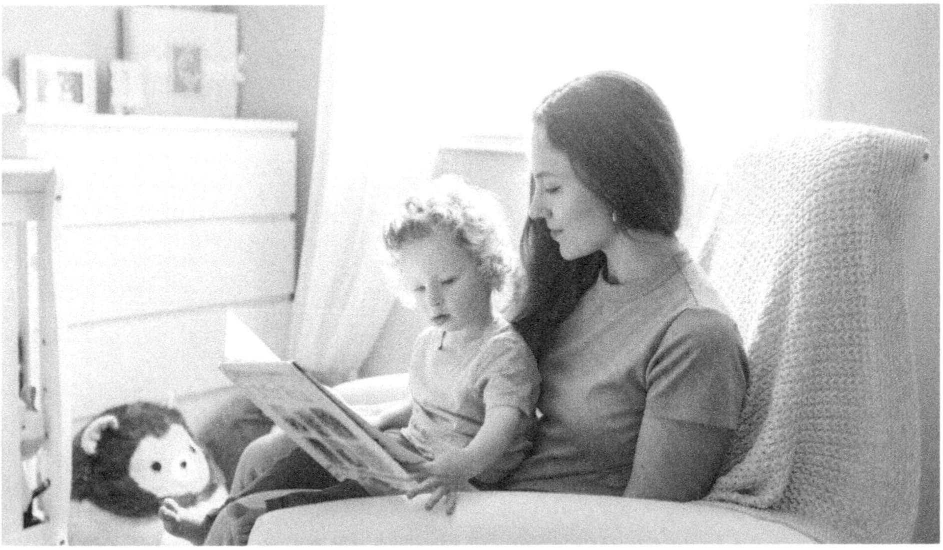

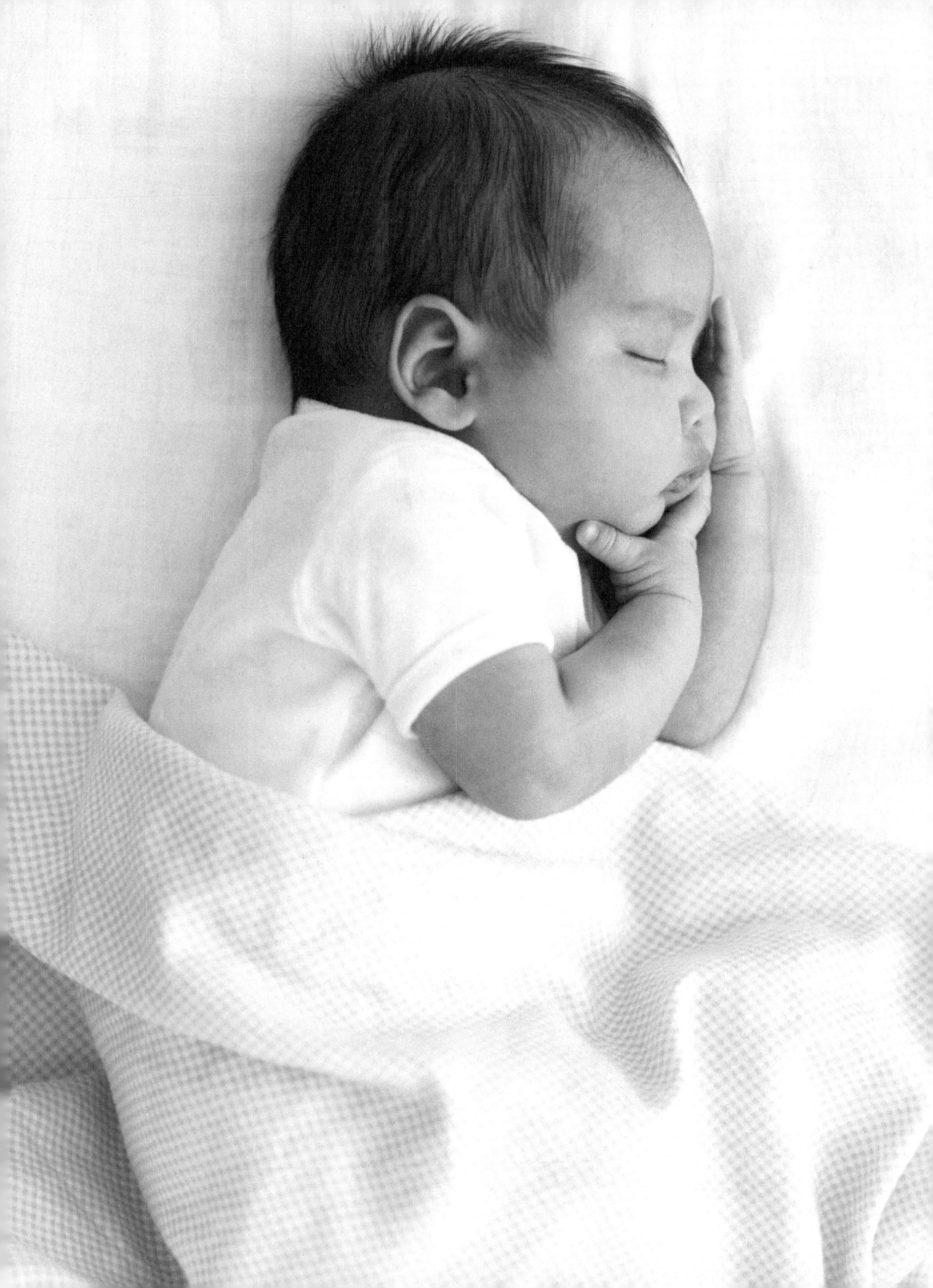

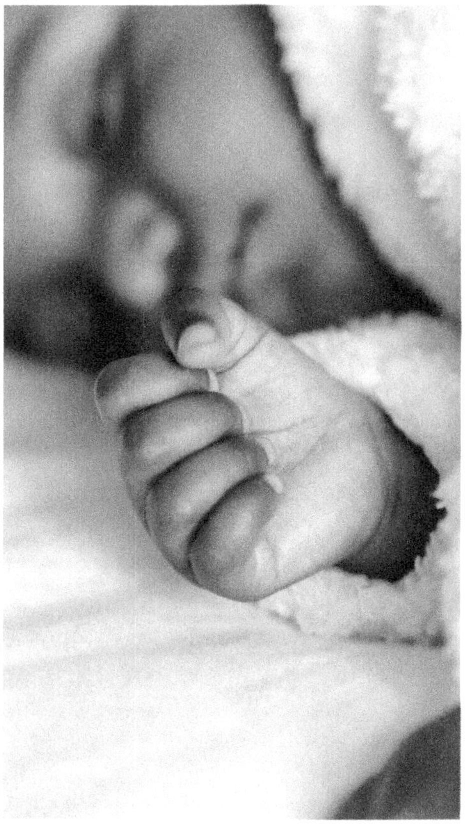
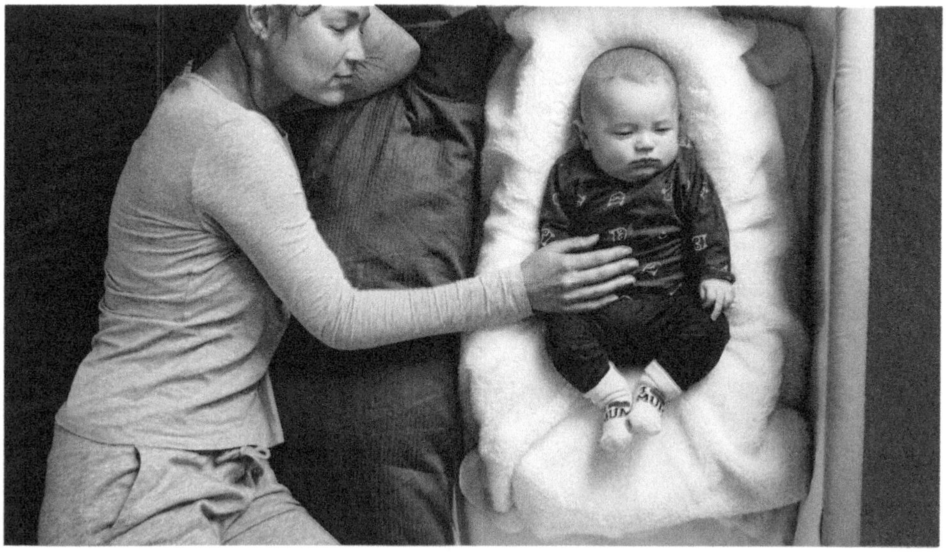
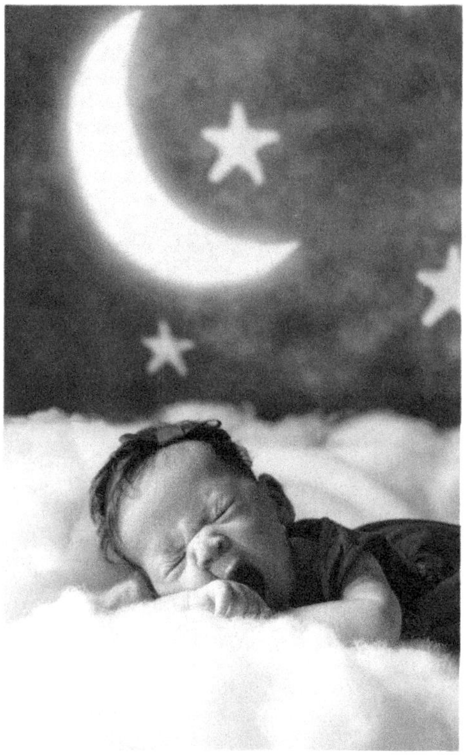
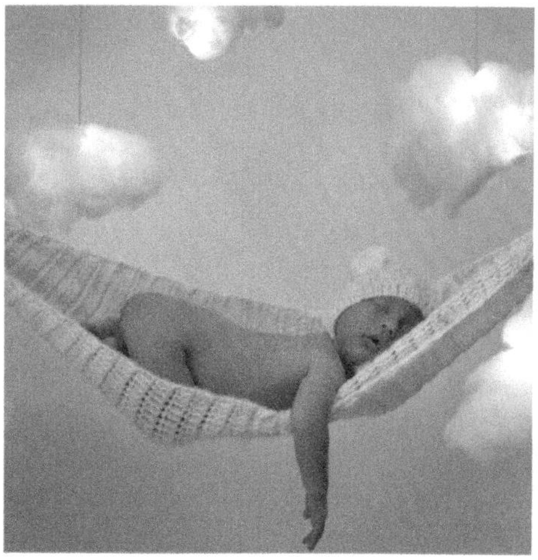
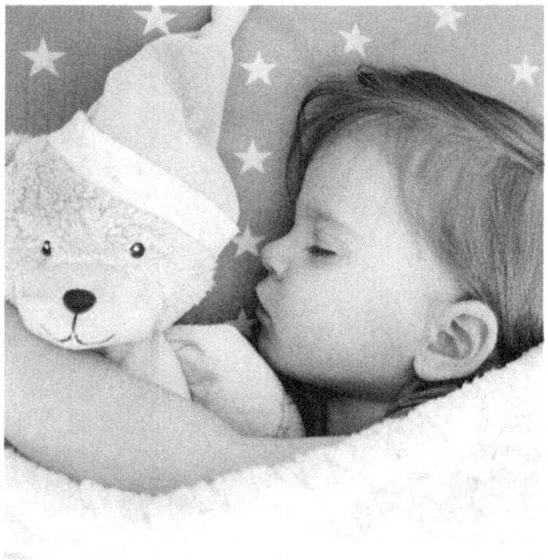
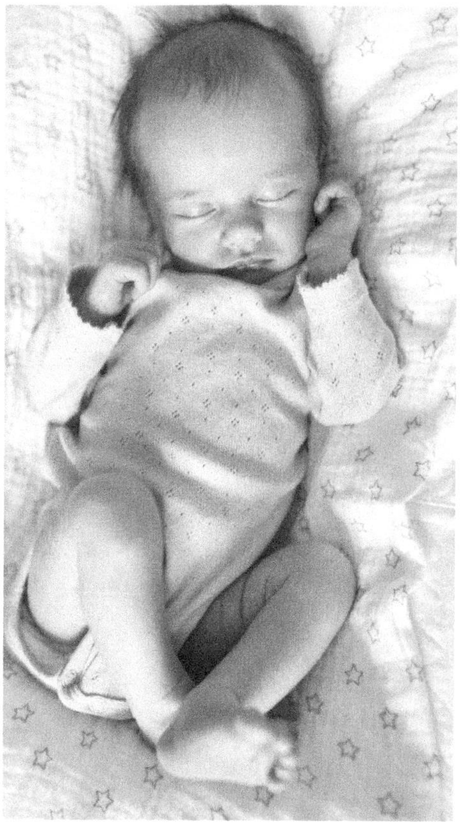
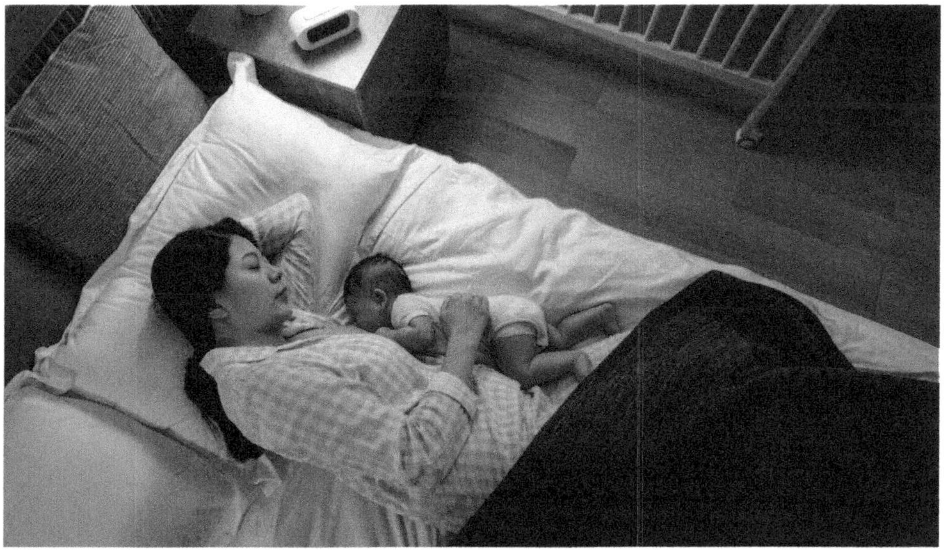

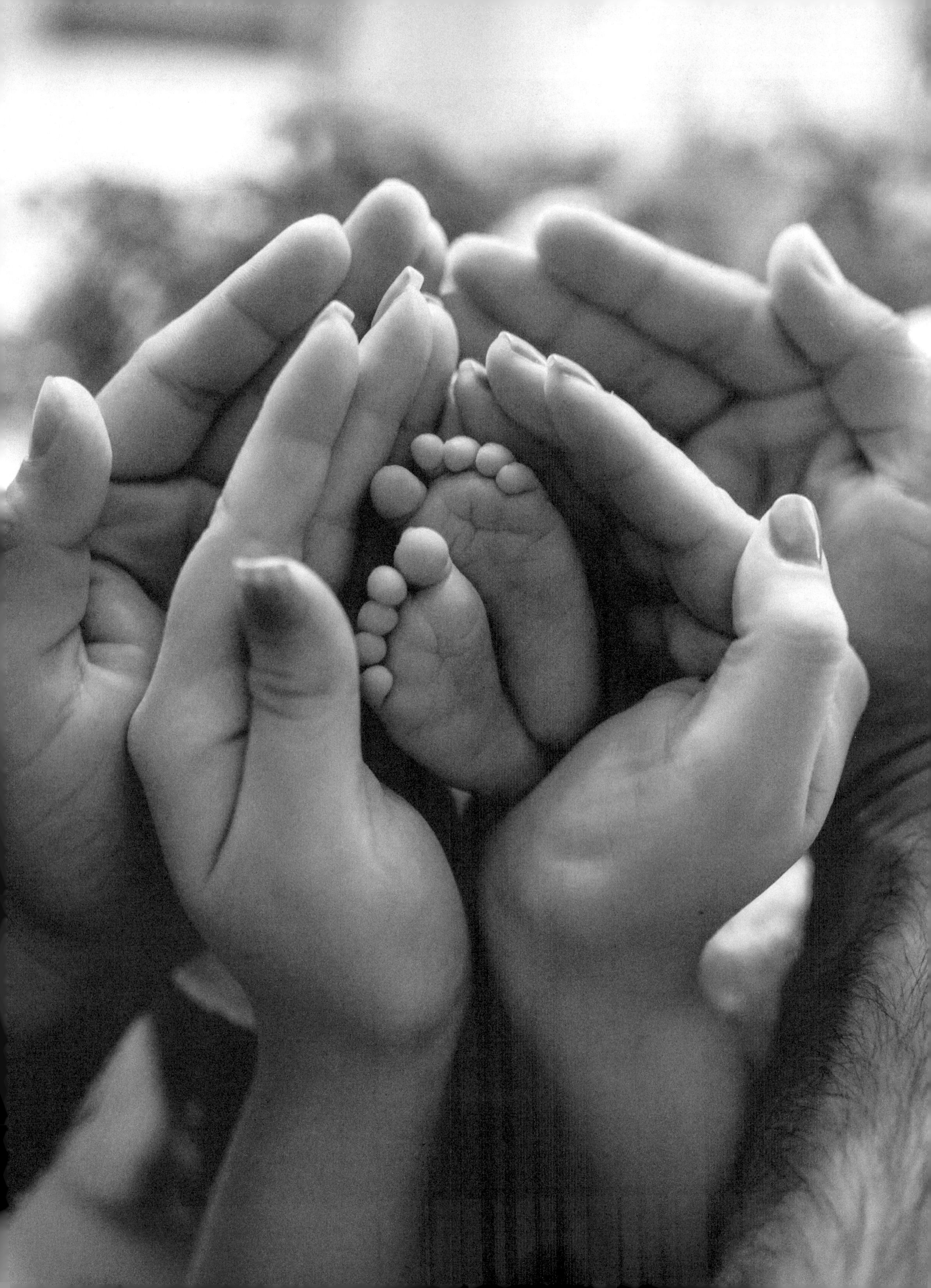